JOHN

SURGICAL AND PRACTICAL OBSERVATIONS ON THE DISEASES OF THE HUMAN FOOT

WITH

INSTRUCTIONS FOR THEIR TREATMENT
TO WHICH IS ADDED ADVICE ON THE
MANAGEMENT OF THE HAND

Elibron Classics
www.elibron.com

Elibron Classics series.

ISBN 1-4021-7029-7 (paperback)
ISBN 1-4212-8350-6 (hardcover)

This Elibron Classics Replica Edition is an unabridged facsimile of the edition published in 1845 by Henry Renshaw, London.

THE

DISEASES OF THE FEET.

SURGICAL AND PRACTICAL

Observations

ON THE

DISEASES OF THE HUMAN FOOT:

WITH

INSTRUCTIONS FOR THEIR TREATMENT.

TO WHICH IS ADDED ADVICE ON

THE MANAGEMENT OF THE HAND.

BY

JOHN EISENBERG,

Author of "Practical Exposition of the Human Foot."

LONDON:

HENRY RENSHAW, 356 STRAND.

EDINBURGH: MACLACHLAN, STEWART, AND CO. DUBLIN: FANNIN AND CO.

1845.

TO

MARSHALL HALL, M.D. F.R.S. L. & E.,

FELLOW OF THE ROYAL COLLEGE OF PHYSICIANS, LONDON; LECTURER ON THE THEORY AND PRACTICE OF MEDICINE AT ST THOMAS'S HOSPITAL,

&c. &c. &c.

SIR,

I have the honour to dedicate this Volume to you.

The extensive practice in which you have been engaged, the valuable information you have given to the world, have placed you in such a distinguished position that your name attached to a work is an honour of which the first medical and surgical authors would be proud. I am indeed rejoiced that this tribute of my respect and admiration has been accepted by you, and that you consider the labours of an humble individual, upon a neglected branch of knowledge, not unworthy your kind protection and consideration.

I am, Sir,
Your obliged and humble Servant,
JOHN EISENBERG.

14 COCKSPUR STREET,
LONDON, JULY 10, 1840.

Vorwort.

In den folgenden Seiten habe ich mich bemüht meine Leser in gedrängter Kürze, doch wie ich hoffe, auf eine nützliche Weise zu einer besseren Bekanntschaft mit sich selbst zu führen; hinlänglich werde ich mich belohnt fühlen, wenn sich meine Bemühungen, durch Linderung gegenwärtigen Schmerzes und Verhütung künftiger Leiden, erfolgreich bewähren.

London im Julimonat, 1845.

Der Verfasser.

INTRODUCTION.

I VENTURE to offer to the public the result of considerable experience in the treatment of the diseases of the feet, with a conviction that the wish to be useful, however humble may be the means, will be fairly appreciated. I do not think that I have given an undue or an inordinate consideration to what has been too often looked upon as trifles. Those who once have suffered from the diseases which are the subject of this volume will readily acknowledge that I have not only laboured upon the more ephemeral annoyances to which flesh is heir to, but they can readily judge, from the excruciating pain they have undergone, that I have nothing exaggerated. The largest portion of society, fortunately for themselves, can form no idea of the usefulness of such a manual as I have drawn up. They have been taught to look upon corns as in themselves so trivial a source of complaint, and so easily remedied, as to be of little moment. In this country especially they have been considered as unworthy surgical skill. In the same manner, fifty years since, attention to the teeth was looked upon as a sort of unnecessary waste of time. The dentist had neither education nor skill; he was looked upon as a mere tooth-drawer, who might be useful in a moment of pain. Now we see men of the highest medical education embark in the profession, and the consequence is, a great improvement not only in the appearance of persons in society, but health is much improved, and longevity is more common. Old people are enabled to masticate their food by artificial means, and thus digestion is more easily and more advantageously performed. But a few years since a horse-doctor was looked upon as an ignorant pretender, and his advice only taken when the hope of recovery of an animal was abandoned. The good sense of a large portion of the community was at length directed to many points connected with the diseases of horses. We have now a Royal Veterinary College, with professors and accomplished men belonging to it, and an experienced man in that branch of knowledge is regarded with respect and esteem. It is not improbable that before any great length of time has elapsed Chiropodists will be admitted to their place in the social system; nor will the hospitals and colleges disdain to receive amongst their teachers men who have studied the diseases of the feet, now unfortunately so little known and so completely disregarded. Beauty of carriage is mainly dependent on the judicious preservation of the feet, and in vain is the body drilled by the dancing master or by the serjeant if the great support of the whole frame be in a disordered state. Personal comfort will be lost without care; besides which, as maladies advance, all locomotion is prevented, and hence a phalanx not only of corporeal but mental sufferings springs up. I trust that those who read my volume will feel that I have sought to add something to the means that we possess of mitigating disease, and that I have not attempted to expatiate upon a subject with which I am not thoroughly acquainted. I have pointed out the great results of personal experience, besides those which I derived from pursuing my studies under competent authority abroad. On the Continent the Chiropodist is estimated as a public benefactor, and has the power of teaching others, and demonstrating such modes of practice as he himself is most familiar with. In every large town in Germany he pays periodically his visit to the different families under his own immediate care. Most of the courts have upon their staff of medical men some Chiropodists; in this enlightened country I am not aware that there is one hospital specially having a professor who devotes his time to the subject.

There are many minutiæ upon which there is little occasion to dwell in a work of this class, which I have necessarily omitted, and I am fully aware that there are repetitions; but they have been unavoidable, because there are opinions which I have advanced which cannot be too forcibly impressed upon those to whom the enjoyment of life's best blessings is not only an object as far as they themselves are concerned, but who would guard the young, and those who are dearest to them, from encountering sufferings which, by caution and attention, may be avoided. The principal subject of my examination has been the affections to which the feet are liable; but I have not confined myself to them, I have ventured upon points which have likewise been carefully studied by me, and on which I trust it will be found that I have been enabled to throw some light—namely, the management of the hand, which scarcely any writer has touched upon. I have attempted to give such original views as presented themselves to my mind; and if, upon mature reflection, I have thought it right to express any opinions which may be at variance with those generally received, I hope that the desire I have had in view, of being useful, will plead my excuse. I have throughout attempted, as far as I could, to write in plain and unadorned language; and when it is borne in mind that I am not a native of this country, and that during the period at which I was pursuing my studies I was at a German university, I entertain little doubt that my efforts will be viewed without that critical examination which even the most erudite and polished performances are sometimes unable to meet. There are very few works, either in the Latin, French, German, or English, upon the subject of my consideration, and I have therefore ventured to add one to the number, which may be found to contain matter that may serve as a guide to those who would hereafter desire to add their own experience, and I shall have fulfilled my anxious desire to be of use to my fellow beings, if I am the means of arresting the attention of parents, of inducing them to take proper precautions, and of alleviating those sufferings to which human nature is unfortunately liable. It would be presumptuous in me to expect that any great success may attend my literary labours, but should I be as fortunate in gaining the kind opinions of my readers as I have been of my patients, by my unremitting anxiety to excel in the profession I have selected, I shall not consider the time I have employed in compiling these sheets thrown away, or regret that I have ventured to become an author.

CONTENTS.

CHAPTER I.

CHAPTER II.

CHAPTER III.

CHAPTER IV.

CHAPTER V.

CHAPTER VI.

CHAPTER VII.

CHAPTER VIII.

CHAPTER IX.

APPENDIX.

THE STRUCTURE OF THE HUMAN FOOT WELL WORTH THE STUDY.

DISEASES

OF

THE FEET.

THE mechanism of each part of the human frame has been acknowledged by every one capable of examining it, to be calculated to excite the wonder and admiration of all intelligent beings. The beautiful adaptation of each organ to perform the function for which it was destined has struck every inquirer into the harmony of Nature; and although in investigating the causes and effects of disease and of decay, we may be baffled in many of our researches, we are permitted to collect together a vast mass of facts which still further inspire a love of knowledge, and an ardent desire to become acquainted with as much as our intellectual powers are capable of acquiring. This curiosity properly stimulated has led to the culture of those sciences deeply important to mankind, which are known under the name of Medicine. A number of the most intelligent members of society have handed down from age to age means by which suffering might be alleviated and life prolonged; but many most important infirmities have been scarcely touched upon, either from the rarity of their occurrence or from their being considered unworthy the attention of men of superior intellect. Amongst the affections to which we are liable, but which have scarcely met the investigation which they require, are those to which the Feet are subject. They have been generally deemed of so trivial a nature as to be unworthy serious inquiry, and they have consequently been consigned to a class of men whose supreme ignorance has thrown obloquy upon those who have both the wish and the power to do good. In the present day we find a large portion of the community, from the highest to the lowest, subject to severe suffering from the inattention of Surgeons to those points, although at the period at which medical science may be said to have dawned, the greatest of the English Physicians, Sydenham, expresses his anxiety that skilful operators should not disdain to devote their attention to this neglected portion of their duties. However trivial may appear the inconveniences which attend upon maladies of the Feet, and however they may be sneered at as beneath the dignity of science, they nevertheless demand that they should meet with attention; and amply will the inquirer be repaid by the information which he must gain, and the power he will possess of being a contributor to the ease, if not the happiness, of mankind. The exquisite beauty of the mechanism of the hand, its influence upon the social, nay, the intellectual happiness of man, has been the theme of one of the first philosophers of the age, and if equal talent and power were devoted to the inquiry and the construction of the Foot, its singular arrangement of parts, its uses in the great economy of nature, we may affirm that it would not afford less subject for ingenious speculation, nor for admiration of Him that framed it. It would require little skill to show that even our enjoyment of intellect, and our capability of deriving from creation around us the best blessings, are mainly dependent upon that organization by which our locomotion is performed, our power "cœli convexum tueri," and to hold that upright form, which essentially distinguishes man from all the living beings which the hand of Nature has so profusely made.

Physiologists have with praiseworthy diligence examined into the anatomy of the integuments of the human body, both with a view to becoming acquainted with the structure and with the uses for which they are destined, but although there has been minute microscopic examination, we find that we are not completely conversant with all the matters connected with them. The interesting investigations pursued both by the late Dr Wallace, of Dublin, and by Mr Judd, have not sufficiently elucidated a subject still wrapt in much obscurity; we have, however, attained sufficient knowledge to explain most of the phenomena which we witness. We find that there are three tissues to which the name of dermoid coverings is given, each performing certain functions necessary to the healthy condition of the body, and each liable to certain deviations from the normal state, which are productive of pain and disorder. The first of these tissues is a membrane, varying in its degrees of thickness, distributed over the surface of the human body, to which the name of epidermis is given: the second is a congeries of vessels from which is constantly issuing a secretion which lubricates the under surface of the epidermis. To this tissue, from its resemblance to a collection of net-work, and from the exudation which is always pouring forth from it, the term rete mucosum has been applied; beneath this is that covering which from its exquisite sensibility, and from its being apparently the natural seat of sensation, has been called the cutis vera, or true skin; its upper surface receives from the rete mucosum a portion of its secretion. Each of these tissues appears to have been considered absolutely necessary for the welfare of the human being; they protect him from the agency of external causes, which would prove pernicious to him; whilst at the same time they enable him to enjoy all those gratifications which arise from the sense of touch so generally diffused over the whole of the external system. The epidermis, a thick layer in most parts of the body, prevents the imbibition into the system of any deleterious matter, and its absence from accident is productive of the greatest mischief. Its abrasion has been known to be the source of danger and of death. The poison of the mad dog is drank in as soon as it is penetrated; prussic acid kills when applied to the skin, when deprived of it. The celebrated Scharinger, of Vienna, having rubbed upon his arm a small quantity of prussic acid highly concentrated, included a small spot where the epidermis was wanting, and instantaneous death followed. A minister in France, under the care of Majendie, was poisoned in a moment by the application of the smallest appreciable quantity of strychnine to a part of the skin which had been denuded of its epidermis.

This tissue resists in a singular manner the ordinary decay to which the human body is subject; it is not unusual, on the discovery of a corpse which has been for years beneath the surface of the earth, to find that the epidermis has remained almost uninjured, and the external appearance of the frame has led to the belief that the usual process to which nature has recourse for the removal of dead animal matter has not occurred, but upon closer examination it has been seen that the epidermis alone presents this appearance. In coffins large masses are found when the rest of the body has decayed away, sometimes the whole of the portion covering the foot is seen apparently in its normal state. The formation of this tissue is not thoroughly understood, but the general impression is that it arises out of the secretion of the subjacent mucous tissue. Its structure has been closely examined; Malpighi, Grew, Lewenhoeck, have been the authorities upon which most anatomists have rested; but upon some of the most important facts there are discrepancies of opinion into which it is unnecessary for me to enter, but which prove how difficult it is, upon a subject apparently easily investigated, and which is interesting to all, to arrive at conclusions satisfactory to us. We are, however, certain that this tissue is formed of numerous laminæ, or scales, which overlap each other, much as do the tiles that protect the upper part of a house. It has even been asserted that the ingenuity with which we roof in the coverings of our domiciles to prevent the action of rain, and of external mischief, is apparently the most insignificant imitation of the structure which protects man's person from the agency of similar inconveniences. The microscope exhibits the epidermis to be much of the same character as the scales which protect fish, and the magnifying power of the hydro-oxygen microscope has unfolded some very curious circumstances which connect themselves with points of importance relating to this external covering. The only object which demands the attention of the Chiropodist, with regard to the physiology of the integument, is as to the manner of its production, for as pressure has been generally believed to be the sole cause of corns, it is necessary for me, in the course of the present treatise, to draw attention to the structure of the epidermis, and also to the tissue, which, lying under the epidermis, is so immediately connected with it, so materially influencing its condition, both in its healthy and its unhealthy state.

The epidermis, if lost, is speedily restored; a scale of thickness is rapidly formed; but its absence, as I have had occasion to mention, may become a source of serious mischief when raised from the subjacent tissue, as is done by vesication. We find it transparent, composed of vascular fibre, and in most instances abounding with lines. Whether actual foramina exist, through which the sensible and insensible perspiration pass, has been the subject of some doubt. It has been asserted that it is transmitted under the scales, which are of exceeding minuteness. Immediately under this scurf, skin, or epidermis, is a tissue, to which the term, from its net-like appearance, of rete mucosum has been generally applied. It appears to be the termination of innumerable capillary vessels, which secrete a mucus of singular character. This is the seat of the pigment which gives the colour to the varieties of the human race. To this the European owes his redness, the Chinese his tawny hue, and the negro his blackness. A portion of this mucus lubricates the upper surface of the cutis vera, and another the inferior surface of the epidermis. It is, generally speaking, of nearly the same thickness as the epidermis, but varies in different parts of the foot. It is in this tissue that, I believe, may be found the first cause of corns, and it is to the inspissation of the secreted mucus, as I shall have occasion to show, that the existence of these annoyances is owing. Under this layer lies the cutis vera, or true skin; it has been considered as a tissue formed of the immediate termination of the nerves and vessels which ramify over its surface. It is the source of sensibility and the seat of touch, and by it sensation is conveyed to the cerebral and medullary masses. It appears, too, to be endowed with the power of imbibition, for any substance may have its peculiar properties conveyed with extraordinary rapidity to the brain, the lungs, the heart, or to the secretions of the body; hence it is that substances rubbed on the skin transmit their power to the stomach, for on the removal of the epidermis and the application of medicinal substances to the subcutaneous tissue we can produce sleep, act upon the bowels, cause vomiting, or give tone and strength to the general system.

It has been erroneously asserted that pressure

upon the epidermis is the sole cause of corns; that its vessels, becoming injured and hypertrophied, throw out a larger quantity of lymph than is necessary; and that the consequence is the generation of layers, which become interwoven. Were pressure the sole cause of corns they would not be confined to so small a surface, they would necessarily embrace a much larger portion of the foot, and we should find the heel, where the greatest pressure exists, the most frequent seat of disease. Some persons are annoyed in a most extraordinary degree by corns, who are the most careful in the selection of their shoes, whilst many who are in the habit of wearing such tight shoes as to be almost incapable of walking, and who seem to wish to resemble, in their incapacity for movement, the Chinese ladies, are totally free from them; besides which, infants have been known to have striking excrescences. There is no doubt whatever that the pain and uneasiness attendant upon a corn are exacerbated by the pressure of a tight shoe, and that instantaneous relief attends a change; but this is easily explained. A new boot sometimes is said to have been the cause of the mischief, whereas the corn has not only long existed, but has formed for itself, in boots that have been worn, a cavity. We constantly find that those who live in towns are more subject to corns than those who live in the country, although the materials of which their boots and shoes are made are so much harder and rougher. It is not at all an uncommon thing for a person who has been afflicted with serious excrescences to lose them altogether whilst in the country, and again to be burthened with them on his return to London. The alteration of structure, wherever corns exist, is of the most decided character. No longer can it be considered as organized texture, for the laws of vitality have altogether ceased within its immediate range; vessels no longer circulate through it their normal fluid; nor does the rete mucosum furnish longer that mild lymph which lubricates the superior surface of the cutis vera, and the inferior surface of the epidermis, but in its place there is an exudation of a serous-like fluid, which rapidly hardens and thickens, layer accumulates upon layer, a corneous substance is formed, which gradually insinuates itself either amongst the muscular fibre, or the minute arterial vessels enter into the softer and spongier parts, assist in giving here and there vitality, and become the source of that exquisite pain which is often complained of by the sufferer. Corns thus developed are more generally difficult of cure, and require all the skill and care which can only be acquired by practice; and he only should venture upon any attempt to cure them, who from long experience is capable of judging by the eye of the exact nature of the difficulties he has to contend with.

That injury done to a portion of the rete mucosum causes the pouring forth of an additional quantity of its secretion; and alteration of its character, from the inflammation produced, may be shown from the singularly aggregated form in which the corn appears. It is almost always in layers, and it radiates from a centre, this point having a larger number of laminæ than any other portion; at first the appearance is simply of hardened pellucid mucus, but gradually different colours are not unfrequently assumed, according to the inspissation of the secretion, and then of the attempt made by the capillary arteries to inosculate; it becomes in the first instance yellow, exhibiting different shades, from the slightest tinge to the deepest hue, afterwards we observe it to be red or brown, and then in the centre a decided black, sometimes surrounded by a complete areola of inflammation, such as may be seen in the incipient chilblain. These changes sometimes follow one another with singular rapidity, at others they are slow, and there is but a very gradual deposition; this will in some measure depend upon the pressure which the surface has to bear, for upon a tight shoe being discontinued, the inflammation of the rete mucosum being put a stop to, there is no fresh addition of secretion, but the moment it is resumed, fresh irritation is set up, accumulation again goes forward, and generally the longer has been the cessation of excitement, the less is the mucous tissue able to bear a new action, and the more rapidly does the corn again increase. We shall find upon an examination of a corn that it is a successive aggregation of layers, the centre of which is denser and harder than any other portion, and although it may preserve for a longer period its pearly appearance, it nevertheless is more concrete than any other portion of its surface. The reason which may be assigned for this is that there is a greater degree of vitality surrounding this point than at any other portion of the superficies. As it is formed like an inverted cone, it is more immediately in connection with the organized portion, and more subject to the action of the surrounding blood vessels. The greater the distance from the point the less of organization exists. The first development of a corn is hence but little painful, and it is only when it has acquired some extent that it becomes annoying. It not unfrequently happens that although the corn has acquired a considerable extent, it has been unsuspected in its growth, for springing from the lower part of the integument, and not from the epidermis, as has been assumed, its approach has been totally unforeseen, and its first announcement has been pain and suffering. It is this which renders an occasional examination of the feet by a Chiropodist absolutely necessary to those who, being predisposed to these inflictions, are liable to have them produced by some exciting cause which has escaped the general observation.

In thus stating that we must well weigh the

anatomy and the physiology of the cuticular system before we ascribe pressure as the proximate cause of the disease, I have no hesitation in stating that it is frequently the predisposing and the exciting cause, and that it is our bounden duty to instil into the minds of those who wish to enjoy the happy privilege of walking free from uneasiness, the absolute necessity there is of giving full play to the muscles of the foot, and fair and proper opportunity for the skin to exhale the perspiration which is naturally poured forth. Tight shoes produce innumerable mischiefs; it is not only the hardening of a portion of the integuments which result from their use, but the capillary circulation is impeded, the muscular fibre cramped, and the nerves kept in a state of irritation, which even may produce a slight febrile condition of the system. How often do we find ladies who have taken but little exercise during the day, worn out by fatigue, and in a high state of corporeal irritation, from the heat of the foot and the sense of tension over the ankle. Even maladies of striking character have arisen out of this cause; and though the same fearful train of evils may not arise from tight boots, as we find from the confinement of the waist by bad stays, yet many are the afflictions which the observant physiologist has known to spring from the anxious desire that arises in the female mind to possess that which from an early period has been looked upon as an attribute of beauty—the small foot. It is not for me to discuss the dangers that arise from any impediment to the capillary circulation, or to show how wrong it is to cause a venous retardation in any part of the system: that I must leave to those who have taken under their own immediate consideration the health of the community, sufficient must it be for me to express my conviction that during the exercise of my profession I have been witness to deviations from the usual state of health produced by the tightness of shoes and of boots; and where I have been called upon in the higher circles of society to relieve by my own treatment the local sufferings, I have occasionally seen the necessity of placing my patient under medical treatment for constitutional maladies, which would not have existed had the feet been allowed to enjoy the functions for which they were destined by the hand that so wondrously has formed them.

The matchless forms of sculptured beauty which the destroying hand of time has left us in the works of the mighty masters of the classic time, exhibit to us the finest specimens of what the foot would be, if allowed its free and uninterrupted action. We are immediately struck with the admirable manner in which it is organized, both for the support of the frame and for motion; its flexibility, its power of action, its form, seem all to have been the result of the examination of the most perfect human models. We see that there have been no artificial coverings, no compression, no restraint; that the gait must have been free, firm, and elastic; that the natural and healthful action of every muscle, tendon, joint, and bone, was fully studied and expressed. There is no stiffness, no contraction of the heel, or the sole of the foot; to the toes are given their proper functions; we see that only the sandal has been worn merely to cover and protect the integument under the broad and expanded foot; there have been no ligatures, no unyielding bandages, no cramping compresses, all is alike free, healthful, natural. We well can comprehend on examining them how the Macedonian phalanx or the Roman Legion performed its long day's march. We can see how the ten thousand Greeks pursued their daily wearying course through the destroying climate of Asia, marching firmly, manfully, alike across the arid sand, the mountain pass, or the flinty plain. We almost are led to the wish to see the European soldier similarly prepared for his toilsome march. Unencumbered with the unyielding shoe, which sometimes becomes in the day a source of greater annoyance than of comfort to him, he would be enabled to undertake fatigue and privations for which he is now totally unprepared. He would find an elastic tread, a firm command over his muscular system follow upon such a plan. He would be capable of making a charge upon the enemy with greater steadiness, and enabled to bear the shock which he is now less capable of resisting. In this respect we should do well to imitate the native soldier of India, who under the English banner has followed a Clive, a Hastings, or a Keane, when the British soldier has almost sunk from the insuperable difficulties which attend wearing all parts of the dress he has been accustomed to do in England, forgetful of the climate in which he is placed.

It is not for me to enter upon the shape and form of the foot and ankle, but the proper development of the latter in early life is much dependent upon the care and attention paid to the toes, on whose surface the presence of corns is a certain cause of alteration of the general appearance of the lower extremity. The toes are seldom objects of much attention to us. We are too often contented with the common attention to cleanliness, and to the length of the nails; all other circumstances pass unheeded by, until our thoughts are compelled to be directed towards them in consequence of feeling some sudden annoyance or actual pain. Such, indeed, is the carelessness with which the subject is considered, that the slightest allusion in society to these important parts of the human economy is considered by many highly indelicate; and even the subject of corns is discussed with such a species of reserve and mystery as to be almost absurd. A well-instructed young lady would shrink back with horror at any mention made of the natural perspiration of the toes, yet of what importance it is to health! and, when checked, to what diseases does it give birth! We may trace one half of the consumptions of this country to cold suddenly applied to the feet, by which the sensible exhalation is checked; and it is not sufficiently impressed upon the mind that when once the regular perspiration from the feet is checked, that it is a matter of the utmost difficulty to restore it. The nightly foot-bath or pediluvium is in vain had recourse to, although the natural instinct of the human mind has shown that this is the best remedy, the reasons for which it is required are overlooked, and the simple warmth it produces is thought to be all that is required. But the experienced Chiropodist can confirm his medical brethren, who ought to be aware that, if the toes do not freely perspire, and even give out an effluvium, some transpiring tissue must take up the excretory duty. The skin is sometimes the auxiliary; sometimes disease is transmitted to it, and those forms of cutaneous affection which baffle the most skilful arise; at others the lungs are called upon to exhale more than in an healthy state they naturally do; and hence spring up a varied host of maladies which owe their origin to inattention to the humbler parts, as they are considered, of the human frame—the toes—but which, in fact, are as important members of the body corporate as are any of the structures of more complicated organization.

The muscles upon which the motion of the foot depend have been beautifully and concisely given by Sir Charles Bell, in his valuable manual, the 'Anatomy of the Human Body.' No words that I could make use of could more adequately convey a precise knowledge of that which dissection shows; indeed, after looking into a vast number of volumes which have issued from the pen of the most skilful anatomists, both here and abroad, I know nothing that could be more intelligible even to the non-scientific reader. I have, however, in the Appendix, made use of a more brief description, from a treatise written by me some time since.

The power the toes have of supporting the superincumbent weight of the human body, is in a great measure dependent upon their anatomical structure; the smaller ones have each three bones, the larger one, two; upon these sometimes rests the whole of the person. What can be more astonishing than the powers of the most celebrated of our danseuses—what evolutions—what movements do they perform upon their toes. We have seen some of them walk the whole length of the stage of Her Majesty's Theatre upon the great toe, balancing the whole of the body with a precision as marked as it is graceful. No faltering, no hesitation, but an onward progress is made upon tip-toe, the whole weight, power, force, and strength of the frame concentrated as it were upon a diminutive bone. The continual pressure does not derange a single fibre; whilst we are gazing at the steadiness with which the position is maintained, a sudden pirouette is made, the whole of the body rotates upon the toe, we are enchanted with the matchless grace displayed, we are loud in our expressions of admiration of the wondrous art of the accomplished dancer, but we forget the marvellous fabric which admits of this extraordinary performance. We may think of the long hours which have been devoted to the acquisition of these powers, we may shower our garlands upon the artist, but we must not altogether forget the hand which made the small organ, upon whose strength so much depends. Our own daily and ordinary motion would be a subject of much surprise and admiration were we to see it made by the hand of the mechanic, and any one who could imitate it would be rewarded for his skill and his ingenuity. As we walk the toes are called into action, we throw the whole weight of our body upon them, especially the great toe; at every step we elevate ourselves upon them alternately with the heel, and bring the centre of gravity of the body perpendicular to the advancing foot thus progressing onwards, preserving a concave state of the sole, and keeping the body in that upright position which is the glory of man, and in which he has been taught that he bears a resemblance to him who formed him. The deformities that arise are generally the consequence of inattention; distortions, malformations, however, present themselves, which cannot now be the subject of consideration.

The lower extremities are with us destined to be confined in leathern cases, sometimes from the knees to the toes; these are made without much regard to the different structure of individuals, all that the most intelligent of the shoemakers of the day think of is the length and breadth of the foot; some of them, it is true, make a last not from the foot but from the boot, instead of modelling the foot, and from thence making the shoe. To this idea we are so much accustomed that we too often buy what we require in the most indiscriminate manner; we go into the first shoe shop that presents itself to our view, and purchase a ready-made pair of shoes, quite satisfied if they are long enough and do not pinch at the sides; the flexibility of the material is little thought of, and still less is any attention paid to the natural form of each foot, for what fits one is supposed to be equally well adapted to all. This is, however, a fearful mistake, for which a thoughtless person has often to undergo great inconvenience, painful annoyance, and even temporary lameness. The great desideratum is to leave the foot to its natural action, to incumber it as little as possible, and not to place it in immediate contact with hard unyielding materials; and, should there be any defects, to have them carefully remedied, or the best means taken to obviate them. If there is a predisposition to corns, there should be more particular attention directed to their position and the circumstances under which they have occurred; hence much suffering may be prevented, and personal comfort enjoyed. To inclose in a leathern prison a tender and delicate foot, is to commit such an act of self-infliction that we are persuaded that, when the mischiefs which result from it are pointed out, few will be so careless or thoughtless as to encounter them, and whatever the dictates of fashion may be, they will be abandoned should they lead to deformity and to pain. It is true that the compression which was formerly the fashion has been mitigated, and young men are no longer employed for half an hour in struggling to pull on a boot in which they were for days to be tortured until the foot was accustomed to its anguish. Still, however, there is much room for improvement, and much cause for reprobation of the practices even of the present day.

The flexibility of leather is altogether overlooked by those to whose management the manufacture is committed, indeed there is no attention ever paid to the subject ; on the contrary, the shoemaker speaks of the durability and of the lasting quality of the article he wishes to recommend. However much pliability would be advantageous, his attention is directed to its capability of resisting external agents ; he thinks nothing of the foot which is to be cased within it ; flexible shoes are, therefore, not to be expected. I should be most happy to have the power of impressing upon the minds of those most interested in the consideration of these matters the absolute necessity of remembering that it is not only the making shoes waterproof that is the duty of the leather maker, but that there are points of infinitely more value. The wrinkles and the indentations which habit makes in an old pair of shoes ought to be some guide; they show what have been the movements of the foot; they point out the attempts which have been made by the foot to accommodate itself; and therefore they ought to be studied by every one anxious to render his workmanship of value. The deep furrows in an old pair of boots are indications not to be neglected, they ought to be examined as well as the marks, wrinkles, and furrows of the countenance are by the physiognomist. The waterproof boots, now so universally prevalent, are to be viewed with much doubt and suspicion, for although they in many instances do what they profess—withstand the influence of the rain, the dew, and the mud—yet they become stiff and hard, and often after a day's exercise are so uncomfortable, that their being impervious is a matter of little importance. They condense, too, the perspiration on the feet, which are often surrounded by a damp moisture that is highly injurious. The stockings often exhibit the effects; a yellow tinge is given to them; they are covered with a disagreeable dew, and look as if they had been dipped in some oleaginous fluid. When the boots are taken off they seem pertinaciously to adhere to the foot, and occasionally an odour is exhaled which is by no means satisfactory to the olfactory nerves. This kind of leather becomes additionally uncomfortable, in every sense of the word, by being placed before the fire; and if, after a day's exposure to the wet and moistness of the atmosphere, the wearer unconsciously places his foot upon the fender before a moderate fire, a disagreeable odour is emitted, the foot becomes stiff, and on examination the following morning it is found to have become exceedingly harsh and rough in some places, whilst cracks have occurred in the natural bends. Under such circumstances probably a few hours will develop a corn that has long been concealed, for a few hours' wear of a pair of modern boots will be sufficient, from similar causes, to produce excrescences quite sufficient to induce repentance, and to enforce a determination to find out another species of covering in preference to that which has been thus injudiciously used. It is true that sometimes the supplest leather may not be devoid of its disadvantages that it wears more rapidly; still, however, it is the bounden duty of every individual closely to examine the materials of which the covering for his feet are composed, and, if possible, to obtain only those that are very soft and pliable.

The three tunics which cover the body having been thus described, and the attempt made to show the nature and proximate cause of the corn, our next object is to ascertain what is the immediate cause of the pain which, sometimes altogether dormant, at length awakens attention, and leads the invalid to seek some relief to sufferings which increase not as the integuments appear to be more or less involved, but under circumstances which do not at all times seem explicable. We have reason to know that fibrillæ, or threads of nerves, inosculate over the whole foot, and anatomy teaches us that each minute artery is itself fed by arteries still more minute, so minute indeed as to escape the eye, and only to be rendered cognizable by the injections which are thrown into the vascular system, and which then exhibit how fearfully and wonderfully we are framed. That great master of our art, Haller, laid it down as a decisive doctrine, that irritability is the property of muscular fibre, sensibility that of the nervous; it is, however, next to impossible to cut off the connexion between the two, for minute nervous fibrillæ intertwine with every muscular fibre, so that the utmost art of dissection could not separate them, and it may be imagined that the nerves form so intimate a union with the muscular fibre that they almost form an integral portion of it, certain it is that the smallest injury inflicted upon the muscular fibre will be felt, and if I may so say, expressed by the nerve in the sensation of pain. Minute as is the injury which is done to the system by the corn, however healthy the condition of the general system may be, it becomes the source of pain the instant a nervous fibrilla is touched. During the first access of the corn there is little or no suffering, because the rete mucosum, attempting to defend the cutis vera from injury, increases the quantity and quality of its secretion, and this for a time shields the nerves; but no sooner is the superincumbent weight greater than can be borne than pain is felt, with its consequences, the sympathy of the rest of the system; when follows a train of alterations which may be said at least fully to develop the nature of the corn. It is the cutis vera where the nervous fibrilla is acted upon, but the rete mucosum and the epidermis become the apparent disease. It is thus in dropsy, the accumulation of water is not the disease, but that alteration in the termination of arteries or of veins by which the fluid is deposited ; and he who believes that by the evacuation of the fluid he does more than afford relief to the system, errs both in his reasoning and in his practice. The vegetable physiologist finds a singular similarity in the development of the external coverings of the plant to that which occurs in the animal kingdom. He finds an epidermis, a cellular tissue, and an inner covering ; and there are certain diseases to which plants are liable which bear a close resemblance to those which affect the human subject. It is not essential for me to enter upon this inquiry, but it would throw considerable light upon many points now buried in darkness, but which some of the French and German physiologists have slightly attempted to elucidate.

The morbid changes which may take place where any of the nerves are wounded, have scarcely been adverted to by any of those who have had the best opportunities of witnessing them, and much surprise would be excited were they to be arranged and classified. It would be clearly shown that the most alarming of them, even to convulsions, lock-jaw, and death, have followed upon the injury which has been sustained by a neglected corn or an injudicious attempt to remove it. I shall have occasion to speak of such events, but I should have been glad if some surgeon had prepared my way by showing to the Profession how regularly spring up, one after the other, a fearful train of symptoms, when an injury, apparently of little consequence, excites the sensibility of the nerve and the irritability of the muscle in a great degree ; life cannot sustain an injury to the system without a struggle, which gives rise to phenomena that require deeper investigation than has been bestowed upon them even by those who most have thought.

CHAPTER II.

No term could be more expressive than the one used by the Romans to designate a corn, and medical authors have very judiciously employed it, for it signifies a small tack driven through the skin, and nothing could more completely answer the description; spina pedum, or the thorn of the foot, which has been occasionally used, is by no means so expressive of its appearance. A thickening of the epidermis is the first apparent source of the corn, I, however, believe that the original seat of the disease is in a nerve under the rete mucosum, or some part of the net-work; this, from some cause not thoroughly understood, becoming inflamed, pours out an increased quantity of secretion, which gradually coagulates and at last indurates; the under surface of the epidermis, partaking of the inflammatory action, pours forth its lymph for self-protection, and gradually a mass of inorganic matter is formed, the pressure of which upon the cutis vera is productive of pain. It has been usual to give the name of root to the inferior portion of this callosity, and hence has arisen the most incorrect theories and corresponding false treatment of corns. For, thinking of the caudex descendens of the vegetable kingdom, those who have been in the habit of attending these diseases, have thought that, by cutting out the hard surface, they were actually putting a stop to the means by which the growth of the substance was fostered. Nothing can be more erroneous than such a doctrine, and nothing more ridiculous than the often-repeated statement of the thoughtless operator, that he has completely eradicated corns, that they will never reappear, because the callus has been cut out. This absurd belief has in many instances led to the great disappointment of the sufferer, and has too often been the cause of the disrepute into which Chiropodists have fallen who have suffered themselves to be deceived by a confusion of ideas, arising out of a foolish employment of terms.

When natural philosophers began to systematize and divide the animal, vegetable, and mineral kingdoms into classes, genera, and species, the medical professors in the different schools of Europe followed their example in the arrangement of disease, and Cullen led the way to a nosological classification, which has become familiar to all the students of medicine, and it has been the aim of those who have wished to combine simplicity with facility of comprehension, to bring together the diseases of organs into such a system as to enable every one to understand it, and to add his own experience to that of those who have already been practically engaged on the subject. It has been proposed to divide the classes of indurations of the integuments of the feet into two genera or families. Corns, or clavi pedum, and callositates ; the first genus embracing four species—clavus durus, or hard corn ; clavus mollis, or soft corn ; clavus sanguineus, or bleeding corn ; and clavus niger, or black corn ; and the second genus comprehending two states—callositas superficialis, or superficial callosity ; and callositas repens, or burrowing callosity. These again may be subdivided into varieties, which it would now be useless minutely to examine.

This arrangement is certainly not objectionable, and there is no man who has devoted his attention to the cure of these maladies who has not seen numerous examples of these different forms ; and though long experience might enable me to point out some additions to this view, I cannot object to receive it as one from which much practical utility may be deduced, and I can have no objection to add my own experience to that of men who have preceded me in the field of my inquiry, yielding to none of them in the anxious wish which I entertain of adding my own stock of information to that of my fellow labourers in the vineyard. The clavus durus, or hard corn, is that which is most commonly known, and it would be a work of supererogation for me to descant upon that which is familiar to most persons; it however is more or less troublesome, according to the locality in which it is fixed, and is developed with more or less pain, which is usually dependent upon the depth to what is called its root penetrates, it sometimes involves the synovial capsule of the joint, or even descends to the investing membrane of the bone, the periosteum, but the degree of pain is not always an indication of the actual state of the stem, whether it be single or many-forked, whether it be flattened or pointed, whether it be horny or soft, the eye of the experienced practitioner can alone detect these variations by the external appearance.

The clavus mollis, or soft corn, is of a somewhat different texture from the hard corn, and this arises generally from its position, for it is most frequently found either between the toes or close to the nails, where the rete mucosum is less strongly developed, and where also there is less opportunity for the exudation upon whose coagulation and concretion the hard corn generally depends. Probably the first suspicion is awakened of the presence of a soft corn by the sensation which is felt of an extraneous body between the toes, and the idea that first presents itself is that a small piece of gravel or dirt has insinuated itself under the stocking; but symptoms of a more marked character soon occur, and the sufferer gradually finds himself a martyr to an affection which at first appears too trifling to be noticed. He soon, however, feels that he has no dormant enemy to contend with, and is compelled, from the sufferings he endures, to have recourse to proper skill for relief; and indeed, should he be tempted, as sometimes has been the case, to remove his tormentor by excision, he produces a state of inflammation and of acute suffering, as will sometimes for a considerable time baffle remedial agency, and has been known to produce such urgent symptoms as to excite fears of a fatal termination. From all that has been collected on the subject, it would seem that ladies are much more prone to this species of attack than men, and of course various reasons have been assigned, and to narrow-soled shoes has been ascribed the frequency of their suffering from this cause; but it in some degree seems connected with profuse perspiration from the feet; and those who are subject to this species of corn have been remarkable for the large quantity of secretion from the pores of the skin, more especially in the immediate neighbourhood of the part affected, but whether this be cause or effect I will not attempt to determine, sufficient is it for me to point out the fact as one that has been observed. A superficial corn is often to be noticed at the root of the nail, which, like the preceding species, is a source of much annoyance, though it is not so liable to produce the same intense agony, unless it takes possession of the little toe, when, from its greater liability to be pressed upon, it often wears an aggravated form, and is a source of much excitement. Were I to point out the various seats of the soft corn, I should be compelled to exceed the limits to which I must necessarily confine myself; it is enough for me to point out those which are of most frequent occurrence. They all run much about the same course, sometimes causing suppuration, and often attended with so high a degree of irritation as to prevent an individual from following his usual occupations, and at any rate compelling him to abstain from exercise, so that not unfrequently a series of inconveniences follow upon the presence of a minute induration, which is deemed by many too trivial for the advice of a skilful man, and is, therefore, too often neglected until suffering brings repentance for the neglect.

The clavus niger is distinguished from the clavus durus and the clavus mollis by the appearance of a small black speck on the early development of the corn. At first it is not larger than the point of a pin; it rapidly, however, enlarges, acquires a remarkable black hue, is perfectly hard, and is difficult of extirpation. A black coagulum of blood is generally found at the base of this corn, which imparts to it its peculiar hue. It is so imbedded in the cutis vera, so surrounded by the papillæ of the nerves, and so intimately connected with the minute ramifications of the arterial system, that its removal is attended with considerable danger; profuse hœmorrhage has followed upon an attempt at excision. This species of corn must not be tampered with, for danger may present itself even where least suspected. It should be carefully borne in mind that nothing but practical experience can justify a man in attempting to treat these maladies; they are by no means so simple as are imagined, and life may be endangered by injudicious treatment. The fourth species, or clavus sanguineus, demands still more caution, for there is a predisposition to hœmorrhage, from which the name is derived. The excessive vascularity of this corn has led some persons to consider that it has differences sufficient to constitute it a genus instead of a species ; but the vessels which apparently supply it with blood, and give the idea of its being organized, do not enter into its substance, but are distributed in such a way as to give rise to this supposition. This corn has usually, from its first commencement, two or three peduncles separate from each other, and in the interstices which divide them blood vessels have so inosculated themselves as to form, with the peduncles, a congeries, from which, upon the slightest cause, blood is poured forth ; there are likewise intermingled nervous filaments, which are productive of considerable pain whilst the corn is attaining its full growth. The blood is generally arterial, of a florid red colour during the first development, but afterwards it assumes a different character, is dark, and may be supposed to have acquired the properties which usually mark venous retardation. Both these last species of corn are liable, in persons of a nervous temperament, to produce considerable constitutional irritation, and symptoms of extraordinary severity are attendant upon improper treatment; and not only are local pain and uneasiness the consequence, but there are many indications of general suffering, owing to the sympathy which exists in many frames, and the facility with which untoward consequences follow upon the derangement of even a part of the body which is unconnected with the great organs by which the actions of life are carried on. Such persons demand more than ordinary consideration, and their disorders require more tenderness of treatment than we are usually called upon to bestow.

Chemistry has been very properly called into aid for the purpose of ascertaining the precise nature of the substance of which the corn is composed, as well with a view of preventing its appearance as with an idea that light might be thrown on its treatment, but little has been the result. It is not found to differ much from that sort of inorganic matter which is secreted in different forms from the human body. The substance has been subjected to aqueous, spirituous, and acid maceration, but with little result. Sulphuric acid exhibits no power upon it; nitric acid softens it; the hydrochloric seems to have more influence, but it does not act for a considerable length of time; some of the weaker vegetable acid produces a slight change, softening it. Left for a considerable time in cold water, little impression is visible; boiling water seems to loosen the adhesion of the particles of which it is composed, but altogether I may say that little or no light has been thrown upon the subject by the labour of the eminent men who have thought that they were useful to society by directing their minds to points which many might not consider worthy serious investigation. There is little doubt that, whilst the corn is still attached to the surrounding organic matter, it is more easily acted upon by heat and by moisture than when removed, and that therefore chemistry cannot furnish us with many indications which may be of actual service. We shall find that a corn which, when the foot was immersed in warm water, was rendered soft and somewhat gelatinous, will, when removed by an operation, become of excessive hardness, and resist the action of boiling water. A corn of cartilaginous texture in appearance has been softened by heat, and apparently so penetrated by water that it has assumed a totally different character, has been unctuous, and almost mucilaginous. Some vegetable bodies, which in early spring abound with hydrochloric acid, produce some slight influence upon the substance of the corn, and hence have been recommended by the humbler classes of society as possessing curative powers. The exudations from several of our indigenous plants have been considered highly efficacious — the celandine, the lactuca virosa, the conium maculatum or hemlock, the milk thistle, have been all used. The delphinium, or stavesacre, which amongst the people is a favourite remedy for all cuticular excrescences, certainly possesses some slight effect, as do the ranunculuses generally. Of these I may hereafter speak.

There is no part of the human foot in which corns have not occasionally been found, both the most delicate and the most hardened portions of its integuments have been thus affected. The soles of the feet, even in their thickest and least sensitive part, have been studded with these annoyances, but the little toe is generally found to be their favourite position, a large portion of it is frequently thus diseased; the outer joint of the great toe appears also to be more commonly infested with these excrescences, under such circumstances are the more ordinary cases which present themselves to the practitioner, and these are the cases which give great annoyance, without probably exciting that excruciating agony which is felt when they appear on other places. They are found under the nail of the great toe, and then are the sources of much irritation; but there are other positions which they assume, and which are sources of extreme misery to those who suffer from them, for instance, the inner portion of the little toe, close to the nail, has been the fruitful cause of such a morbid condition, that the whole frame has partaken of it, and I have had occasion to relieve an apparently broken-down constitution, by means so simple, yet so efficacious, as to be looked upon rather as a ministering angel than an ordinary observer of the effects which may spring from the humblest means. The roots of the nails have been occasionally the seats of corns which have produced a high degree of inflammation and tumefaction, these have been ascribed to accidents, nay even to a gouty diathesis, whilst the original cause has been overlooked, because little or no pain has attended their development. The three little toes are indiscriminately diseased; some persons exhibit a peculiar idiosyncrasy in this respect, and in families will be found a striking predisposition to having this portion of the integuments of the foot in an unhealthy state. The soles of the feet, and the heels, often exhibit excrescences, varying in the intensity of the symptoms they display; sometimes only those of annoyance, at others of absolute pain. I should much extend my work were I to enter minutely into the appearances which have presented themselves to me during my extensive practice; but I would observe to the student that he must not be surprised at the position and extent of some of the masses which he will from time to time have occasion to see; he must bear in mind that the deviations from the ordinary course of nature are not numerous, but that from the facilities of witnessing the varieties he possesses, he will see so many as to lead to an impression that they are more common than they really are.

The first idea which naturally presents itself to those who are suffering from pain of any kind is instantaneous relief, and many are most willing to allow the "fons et origo mali" to remain, and again to be the fruitful offspring of pain, rather than submit to any additional suffering, even for the sake of altogether eradicating the exciting cause. Thus do we often find a person suffering from the acutest agony of the tooth-ache, who, when made aware of the actual decay of the tooth, and the utter impossibility of preventing a recurrence of the agony, if it be at the moment relieved, shrink from undergoing the only operation by which he can be permanently restored to ease, and seeking palliatives, which doubtless for a time afford some cessation, but cannot altogether put a stop to the disease. It is generally first necessary, even in acute disorders, to examine whether we possess means by which we can alleviate the suffering, and sometimes gain time, and give the system, which has suffered from sympathy, time to recover. In the cure of the disordered state of the feet we must oftentimes devote as much consideration to the means of palliation as well as to those of cure, and we shall find that we often gain reputation from the public, and estimation in the eyes of our patients, from affording them momentary ease as much as from the ultimate cure of the disease. We are in most instances precluded from administering many of those remedies which the skill and knowledge of the medical man enable him to avail himself of in the more aggravated forms of disorders. We shall seldom find, unless indeed the case is one of great urgency, that our patient is willing to apply to those narcotics which affect the general system, for the purpose of affording him relief to a local malady, distant from any important point. He who would submit patiently to a dose of opium, of hemlock, of belladonna, or of stramonium, for a tooth-ache or for an ear-ache, would not be induced to try their effects when the cause of his suffering was seated in the foot, and thus are we deprived of the assistance of some agents of considerable power as palliatives; on the other hand, the confidence of the public is so much abused by a class of self-educated and self-extolling practitioners, who pretend to have discovered infallible means of preventing diseases such as we have described, that innumerable difficulties surround the subject. Specifics for all the ills of life have been discovered daily and hourly, if the public press is to be taken as our guide, for not a sheet issues from the press, but amongst the advertisements will be found the bold assertion of some loud proclaimer of his power, and more especially in the department to which I have devoted my attention; plaisters, ointments, liniments, lotions, are all brought before the astonished world as possessing infallible power. The maker of these nostrums wraps in becoming mystery his discovery, he obtains a patent for it, he signs his own autograph upon the stamp; there is necromancy, witchcraft, and marvellous power in everything he propounds. He has never been known to fail, according to his own assertion, and what chance has he who has devoted his life to inquiry, has honestly to confess that the deviations of nature surpass his expectations, that her ways are often inscrutable, and that all he can do is to study to learn and to attempt to cure, without professing that every malady is subjected to his superior skill.

Most urgently do I recommend those who are afflicted with corns, however harmless they may seem, however easily removed, never to have recourse to the knife. They may be assured that though there may be a vast number of instances in which no bad consequence has attended upon this operation, yet there are so many and such serious events which have arisen out of it, that no one who has a regard for his own comfort and safety should venture upon it. One sad termination outweighs a whole catalogue of fortunate extirpations. I strenuously recommend those who, suffering from corns, are anxious for relief, never to have recourse themselves to the penknife, to the razor, or even to the scissars, but to place themselves as early as possible under the management of some one who has long been skilled in their cure. They will find temporary and sometimes permanent relief, if the affection be but commencing, from plunging the foot in a hot pediluvium, pouring in from time to time hot water, and keeping it steadily immersed at least half an hour. The foot should then assiduously be rubbed for a considerable length of time with a dry rough towel, the friction need not be confined to the immediate surface of the corn, but rather on the integument immediately in contact with it. In the greater number of instances this process will be followed by the loosening and extraction of all the corneous substances; there will be neither pain nor uneasiness left; the sleep will be uninterrupted by any disagreeable sensation, and though the corn may, and most probably will, return, it may again be removed in a similar manner, and should the exciting cause be avoided, there is little doubt that an ultimate cure may be obtained; this, however, is somewhat difficult, and it is too often found that, after a short time, it occupies precisely the same ground that it did before; nor can it altogether be extirpated but by the aid of an experienced practitioner. As I have observed, never should the apparently simple appearance of a hard corn lead to the use of the knife by the patient, for, although there may be nothing from which any bad result could be anticipated, no external characters which give the least indication that evil will be the consequence of a meddlesome practice, yet the most serious consequences may result, and when too late there will be cause for the deepest regret. If I appear somewhat tedious on this matter—if I have been guilty of repetitions—I trust that I may be excused for an earnestness and an anxiety on a subject which I conceive of more importance almost than any rules I may lay down. It is a maxim which I would have a starling taught to repeat; it is a sentence which should be repeated in the ears of every sufferer from corns; it is a voice which should be echoed back upon every occasion—Do not use the knife to your corns! If after such a warning there should be any venturesome enough to neglect it, the danger must be on their own heads; but the repentance will come too late.

I am not fond of giving cases, for I am sorry to find that every empiric who practises any branch of the medical profession fancies that the true avenue to employment is to narrate extraordinary cases, whether they are founded on truth or not, because he fancies that people will see something in what they read which may remind them of their own suffering; but I cannot pass over an opportunity of referring to what occurred during my residence in Edinburgh, and which could not fail to make a considerable impression upon the minds of the highly-polished inhabitants of that city. The lady of one of the most distinguished Professors there had a corn between the toes, which had been the source of much suffering. She cut it with some sharp instrument—blood followed; after this she went into society, and for some days had apparently forgotten the circumstance, when violent pain came on. She preferred sending for her own surgeon, who is one of the most distinguished professors of surgery in Scotland, but he unfortunately considered such an ailment too trivial for his consideration; he passed a sharp instrument, and death was the almost immediate result. This was attributed to the mortification which it was said had been slowly advancing from the moment of her attempt to cut it. I was fortunate enough, at the same time, to be in attendance upon the lady of a distinguished physician residing in Abercrombie place, who had also been rash enough to use the penknife, and to produce mischief for which she anxiously sought my advice in consequence of the former case, and I was eminently successful. I will only allude to the case referred to in the memoirs of the Duchess d'Abrantes; it will be seen in the second volume. I could refer to a vast number of examples, if I thought it necessary to add to the testimony which I here bear to the sad results of using the knife.

The most appalling spasms, convulsions terrible even to behold, and lock-jaw, have attended on the wounding a branch of a nerve by a common penknife, hœmorrhage scarcely to be arrested. The two species I have described under the designation of clavus niger and of clavus sanguineus, least admit of being tampered with; let the appliances be what they may, let the skill be great, still no blood is to be produced from them, until the constitution has been duly prepared, until every advantageous circumstance presents itself. It is not difficult for any person who is determined to acquire the art to enable himself by the assistance of a proper instructor to eradicate corns;

but, like every other species of knowledge, it is to be gained by diligent practice. It is, however, a considerable length of time before a person, however assiduous he may be, is fitted for all the anomalies which present themselves. In attempting to describe the plan to be pursued, I am aware how difficult it is; but there are certain hints which I would throw out for the guidance of those who would commence the manual operations in which I have been for a series of years engaged, and to perform which, with dexterity and success, has demanded on my part considerable labour, observation, and anxiety. No one, however fortunate he may have been in acquiring the confidence of the public, can altogether divest himself of anxious fears when about to commence any operation on which the welfare of a fellow-being is dependent, and I can conscientiously assert that I have at all times exerted myself to the best of my ability to give relief immediately, and that in recommending the abstaining from any operation, it is from a feeling that it would not be attended with success. I have always attempted to maintain self-possession and calmness during the whole of a manipulation, whatever might present itself of unexpected difficulty; and I have been happy enough to have escaped those dangers into which others have fallen. My own plan, which I would recommend to others, as best calculated to ensure success, is to place myself in such a position near the window that the light may fall upon my right hand. I prefer the broad clear daylight, but of course am often compelled to accommodate myself to circumstances. Immediately on a line with myself is placed my patient on an ordinary chair, somewhat higher than my own; his left foot is placed upon my right knee, or his right foot upon my left knee; I am thus capable of carefully examining the seat of the disorder.

Near me are placed, so as to be immediately within my grasp, whatever I may require, or the remedial agents of which I expect to stand in need. I generally find some magnifying or microscopic glasses of great utility to me, often enabling me to ascertain, with great minuteness, objects which might otherwise escape attention.

The removal of the corn is to be considered the great object which the operator is to have in view; he is to detach from the subjacent tissue every portion of the extraneous substance which lies imbedded, and, as may well be imagined, in many instances much time elapses before the different stages into which the operation is divided are concluded, and there must be occasionally such shifting of the mutual positions of the Chiropodist and his patient, as may allow the former every facility for carrying out his object; but each change should be slowly carried out, and no hurry of any kind suffered to throw either party into an uncomfortable position. It sometimes occurs that the elbow must rest upon the patient's knee, and both parties must maintain their steadiness, otherwise a slip of the instrument might occur, which might produce some degree of inconvenience; sometimes the hand must be used where the very minute portions of the indurated mass require to be removed; indeed it is sometimes better to avoid the use of any instrument whilst the loosening of the integument takes place; but these are minutiæ into which it may not be necessary for me to enter, but which are to be acquired by practice. It must be borne in mind that the manipulation which is sufficient for one corn is not sufficient for another, and that so many intermediate varieties from complete adhesion up to slight attachment exist, that it would be irrelevant to describe each; it must also be borne in mind that occasionally there are shreds of indurated skin which are not necessary to be cut, and which would produce pain were they to be needlessly meddled with. It would likewise be trespassing too much on the time of my readers were I to enter upon the positions necessary, and the exact nature of the operation to be performed according to the situation of the corn, whether upon the great toe, the little toe, or the sole of the foot,—each requires some little study to accommodate the operation to the state of the patient. The paring away of the hard induration without the dissection is sometimes necessary to be effected before any attempt at taking out the roots, and the operation may demand more attention, especially if there be much tumefaction and tenderness present, although these symptoms, generally speaking, need not interfere with the process for their relief. The most certain and efficacious plan is to examine the condition of the part on which the operator has been engaged about a week after this sitting. He then is enabled to form a judgment as to his complete success; he will see whether the vacancy that has been made by the extirpation has been filled up by a healthy process; whether the rete mucosum is again pouring forth a secretion which will again indurate and prove a nuisance to the unfortunate patient. Watching the progress of the efforts made by nature for the reproduction of parts that have been destroyed is always one of the most interesting occupations of the physiologist, who often enjoys opportunities of studying a most important leaf of the book of nature. The operation which is set up under such circumstances, as well as those to which I have directed attention, is one of considerable importance, and demands the careful observation of the Chiropodist, who is sometimes called upon to hasten it, or at others to detach unnecessary portions.

However skilful the manipulator may be, no task can be more difficult than the description of an operation, or the precise laws to be attended to when it becomes necessary to have recourse to instruments. It is only practical experience that can be the guide, and it is only the well-accustomed eye that knows the precise moment at which such interference is necessary as may lead to the ultimate well-doing of the patient. A long series of years, a vast number of cases, must found the groundwork on which both theory and practice must rest. In vain will the most accurate language convey the ideas of the observant man if, besides that, there is not the tact and judgment which are only to be acquired by having the attention constantly fixed on a subject, and the readiness which can only be attendant upon habit. It is a well-known fact that everybody fancies he is equal to the cutting his own corns, notwithstanding the numerous instances in which the most disastrous events have followed upon this self-confidence, and there is no man, however ignorant he may be, who does not indulge in the flattering idea that he has only to announce himself to be a Chiropodist to be at once gifted with the knowledge of an intricate art, and to be capable of exercising it not only with perfect safety but with certain success. A few fortunate trials, where there has happened to be only the common-place and ordinary affections, give him the sanguine hope that he has at length found out the avenue to fortune, and boldly does he proceed in his path, until he is suddenly arrested in his onward career by some unexpected difficulty. In an unadvised moment, elated with his sudden good fortune, he has carelessly plunged his knife into one of those apparently unorganized corns in which, unfortunately for him, are numerous ramifications of minute arteries, somewhat more deeply seated than he in his philosophy had dreamt of: a sudden hæmorrhage occurs, he is astonished at the unforeseen catastrophe; he finds, on a more minute inspection of the excrescence which he has so unceremoniously incised, that the tumuor is more circumscribed than he has been in the habit of witnessing; that it has a more spongy substance; that here and there red specks may be traced; both the operator and the patient have reason to congratulate themselves if the only symptoms that follow are painful tumefaction and high constitutional irritation, for fatal events have often sprung from such attempts. I will not attempt to paint some of the scenes which have presented themselves to me. I will confine myself to holding forth a solemn warning to those who, with matchless effrontery and shamefaced daring, attempt to enter upon the practice of an art which demands caution, prudence, and above all serious reflection, before it is attempted to be followed. There can be no objection to reasoning based upon experiment, but an unfortunate patient is not to be made the means of acquiring information. He who attempts to relieve others should have studied under the guidance of one who has already attained knowledge, and there can be no earthly excuse for rashness and ignorance. It is not a scalpel or a knife that are to be used, but there are instruments necessary for different manipulations into a description of which I cannot enter, because they are not to be thoroughly understood without some examples of them, and diagrams exhibiting the precise manner in which they act. Each Chiropodist has his own favourite instrument; some excel in the use of one, whilst another places confidence in one of his own construction. I have the firmest reliance on those which I myself invented, to which long habit has accustomed me, and I fearlessly assert that they would be found by any one who is anxious to acquire excellence in the art, the best that have been invented. At the same time I am most willing to do justice to others, who have with great assiduity and labour brought to perfection manipulatory powers, in which they have with justice perfect confidence. It is sometimes necessary to be enabled to scrape the surface of the corn, to pass beneath it, to elevate it, to lay hold of it, and extract it from the layers in which it is imbedded; all these different operations require their own peculiar instruments. They are to be handled each in its own manner; the hand should therefore be dexterous, light, and flexible, no stiffness of joint, no thickening of the palm of the hand; a quick eye and great steadiness are demanded. There must be no flurry, no haste, no exhibition of doubt or apprehension; calmness and coolness are necessary to the perfection of practice. The operation once commenced must be steadily persevered in, unless cause exist to wait for a time, as is the case if the least quantity of blood is poured forth; this should always prevent any further step, for whilst it may be looked on as somewhat of an unfavourable symptom, it precludes the possibility of seeing what is to be done, or what has been already effected. It has been my good fate, out of above eighteen thousand cases, not to have three times produced blood. It is possible in every case to avoid the smallest bleeding, and it may be considered an untoward event wherever it occurs. The skilful operator avoids it; he neither produces pain nor bleeding, but carries on his work without injuring any part with which he is compelled to come into contact. All the ramifications of the corn are to be diligently searched for; there is to be no superficial passing over any minute branch or stem; there is to be the greatest delicacy, tenderness, and gentleness in every attempt to remove any of the means by which the adhesion is affected. Should there be a suspicion that these adhesions are deeper seated than usual, it is generally proper to suspend for some days any further proceedings: but to give directions on this point is almost impossible, for nothing but long experience can sufficiently give the proper knowledge of what is to be done; caution, however, should always be the safeguard of the practitioner and of his patient.

Both immediately before and after the operation others generally recommend the immersion of the foot in hot water; this measure generally does great harm, especially to the tender foot, the parts immediately around the corn swell and inflame. I am no advocate for the employment of any of those boasted remedies which have been loudly praised as capable of acting upon the induration, and of preparing it for dissection. I have no objection to friction with flannel, but not with hard substances, which many are extremely partial to; amongst these are the pumice stone, the scuttle fish, sand paper, and even rough files. Considerable injury has followed upon their indiscriminate use, and although there may occasionally be circumstances in which they may be properly employed, yet, generally speaking, they do more mischief than good. It is very difficult to confine their use to the mere induration, and the surrounding integuments arc liable to be irritated by them. Some balsams and tinctures have been much spoken of by the older writers on the different excrescences, but modern practice has very judiciously excluded them from their insufficiency to produce any good effect. The radical cure is more dependent upon surgical than upon medical means; and although I should gladly avail myself of any of the suggestions which have been made from time to time for the relief of these maladies, yet I have found no good reason to place faith in any of them. Many are the hints thrown out by our old herbalists in their quaint language as to the powers of some of our indigenous herbs, and certainly in one or two instances their recommendations have apparently had some slight success, but they are better adapted for those slight cases which are benefited by the removal of pressure than for any of those more serious ones which are likely to engage the attention of the practitioner. Amongst the herbs of which they have boasted there is one which certainly has some slight influence upon corns, and is a great favourite amongst the popular writers on corns—it is the common house-leek, the sedum murale. This herb, which is found growing on the tops of old garden walls and upon the roofs of houses, has a leaf of considerable thickness, owing to the large quantity of cellular tissue between its upper and lower lamina, in whose interstices is found considerable juice, which abounds with hydrochloric acid in a free and uncombined state, which may easily be shown by means of nitrate of silver, for it speedily enters into combination with the silver, forming that which is commonly known under the name horn of silver. Owing, doubtless, to the presence of the acid, the juice acts upon the indurated mass, softening and destroying the surface, but leaving the lower parts as great a source of mischief as ever, and sometimes converting the corn into a more hardened mass than it was before. Those who have tried the remedy seem decidedly averse to its repetition; from my own experience I have nothing to observe, having collected from others what I have now said.

The great object in the sole of the shoe is

hardness, and the flatter and more even the better. Many persons have most injudiciously recommended that holes should be perforated in cork soles and false bottoms, with a view of giving room to the corn, and thus to prevent pressure. To this I most decidedly object, for the result is generally irritation and inflammation of the surrounding integument, and a constant state of indescribable annoyance. The sole of the shoe should be made of one solid substance, and not of three laminæ, as is generally the case ; for the innermost produces swelling and considerable uneasiness of the surface, than which nothing is more hurtful. Few people pay proper attention to these points, and shoemakers follow their own inclination, and generally tell their customers that a few days will make the boot stretch and the foot will settle down. When we reflect that many diseases in the head are the consequences of the compressed circulation in the foot, it is a matter of astonishment that so little attention has been paid. It has happened not unfrequently that a person suffering from a corn in the sole of the foot, or some soreness of the integument, has fancied that relief was to be obtained by a soft lining placed within the sole of his shoe, and has had recourse to one of the cork soles covered with lamb's wool which are sold in the shops. He has worn it for two or three days, when, to his inexpressible surprise as well as sorrow, he has found not only darting pains across the footstep, pain in the back of the great toe, but even that disease which I am about to describe—the bunnion—has threatened him with all the affliction that attends upon it. "Incidit in Scyllam cupiens vitare Charybdim," he has expected to avoid one mischief and has fallen into another even worse to bear. Strenuously would I recommend, therefore, that no fancied relief from soft, warm, yielding materials, should tempt him who suffers to try its effects; he will bitterly regret it, and then the advice which I have offered may recur to his mind. It is from my own experience, moreover, that I offer my recommendation, for others have given opinions the reverse of mine, and those who have followed them have uniformly told me that they have to their sorrow found they were misled by misrepresentations which sprung from theory, but were not based on practice.

It not unfrequently happens that a person who comes up to London, although much accustomed to pedestrian exercise, has scarcely trod our well-paved streets a week, before he discovers that his change has at least been productive of one unexpected annoyance; he finds for the first time that he had corns, to which he did not dream that he had the slightest predisposition. On the other hand, a person who has always breathed the air of the great metropolis, who has daily taken his walk from the West End to the City, no small distance every day, on going into the country finds in a few days that he must abandon the luxury of walking, for he has for the first time become subject to the painful inconveniences of which he has heard so much, but fortunately felt so little. Thus we find that an alteration in the tread of the foot is a frequent source of annoyance. The simple change from a rough to a smooth surface; or, on the other hand, from the smooth to the rough, demands an imperceptible difference in the motion of the muscles and their integuments, and the joints seem to attempt to relieve themselves, for near them the rete mucosum commences that series of action which is the first cause of the induration of the integument. This may be obviated by the use of a different shoe—a more elastic one is demanded for the pavement than for the hard road, for which a thicker material is necessary. Amongst the subjects which have been frequently discussed is the singular state of corns just previous to wet weather. The common expression, "we are about to have damp from the shooting of my corns," has naturally led to some remarks; and there can be no doubt whatever that different states of atmosphere act upon the integuments of the human body. Electricity has a wondrous influence both upon body and mind, and in damp weather we are constantly giving up the natural electricity of the system. For such is the tendency to a general equilibrium of caloric and of electricity, that bodies are continually in a state of change, either giving off or receiving them. One of the learned physicians of the day has instilled into the minds of the public the advantages of wearing silk next the skin, for, as it is a non-conductor of electricity, it keeps within the body that which has been generated there. We shall find that the lower extremities are remarkable for the influence produced upon them by atmospheric changes. Few things are more striking than the appearance of the large sparks of electric fire and the loud crack which occur when a silk stocking is pulled off. In the dark the peculiar blue light is singularly visible,—a long train of fire seems to issue forth, and not unfrequently this is attended with a peculiar tingling sensation. Persons of a nervous temperament more particularly exhibit this phenomenon, delicate females more especially; and there seems to be some connexion with maladies of the nervous system generally. We find such persons more than usually listless, given to yawning, and incapable of following any pursuit with vigour. They are liable to glandular swellings, and to attacks of inflammation of the tonsils or throat, showing what a sympathy exists in different parts of the body. Many such are afflicted with painful corns, singular as such a fact may seem; every medical practitioner, upon looking over his roll of patients, will find confirmation of it. But the phenomena of disease are, as the inquirer into that branch of philosophy acknowledges, connected more or less with hygrometrical facts. In a work to which we have elsewhere alluded, as one from which most of the knowledge which practitioners had of corns was derived, is a very curious and at the same time a remarkably well drawn up view of the effects of the atmosphere upon the corn, exhibiting the influence of its pressure upon the system generally, and upon these small excrescences particularly. The weight of atmosphere upon the human body is equal to two thousand two hundred and sixty pounds, and therefore the pressure upon each square inch amounts to nearly nineteen pounds; if we then take the proportion of the foot upon which the weight of the atmosphere is more or less increased, we shall find that there is under certain circumstances such increased pressure upon the integuments, that the subjacent parts must feel the full force. To those who have known what the simple exhaustion of a small quantity of air in a cupping glass effects as to the sensation of weight on the body, there can be but little difficulty in comprehending what changes may result from the weight of the atmospheric air upon the corn, driving it into the subjacent tissue with considerable force, such even as to affect the minute capillary vessels, and the small nervous fibrillæ, which exist to such an extent over the greater part of the foot. This is a question, however, into which I have no inclination to enter; sufficient is it, that those who are tormented with corns should occasionally be reminded of their presence, that they may seek those means of relief which are afforded them. I do not pretend to be enabled to account philosophically for the effects of heat and cold upon them, but to point out that it is necessary to take some precautions as soon as they become troublesome; and that those who are negligent, because there is no immediate bad symptom, may suddenly, even from change of weather, be laid up, and prevented from following their usual avocations. Months, nay years, may sometimes pass by, and trifling inconvenience only arise; but as age creeps on, as the system becomes less capable of self-restoration after disease, as the integuments become harder, so is there greater difficulty in eradicating or curing these complaints. The young should not allow them to exist, for they will grow with their growth, and will oftentimes impede them when most they are anxious for activity and exertion. Those who are advancing in life should bear in memory that their defects are soon aggravated, that wounds are more difficult to heal, that the renovating powers lose their vigour as time creeps on, and therefore none should delay. They will find that they are destined, like the rest of the race of man, to some of those evils which beset us; fortunate indeed is it that they are capable of being remedied; and, as the means lie within our grasp, they are not to be neglected, but every effort made to combat them, and thus pass our time in comfort and ease, when so little may disturb our most anxious searches after repose and tranquillity.

The summary of long experience in the management of corns I would willingly give in few words, but there are many points which must be dwelt upon, for without sometimes expatiating on them they are likely to be speedily forgotten, but I should most strenuously impress upon the minds of all that the earlier attention is paid to a corn the better; the moment it excites the attention it ought to be attended to by some experienced person, for to what extent it may arrive without due attention it is difficult to say. If it is seated upon a joint it ought not for a moment to be neglected, for it is probable that it will soon become an impediment to exercise of any kind, besides which it is much more likely to return if it arrive at a certain stage. When arrested in its progress in its early stage it will most probably never again be seen, but relapses are more likely to occur if situated there. Although cures are sometimes spontaneously produced, yet they are rare, and however complete may appear the cure, yet at a most unexpected moment the corn may recur without there being the slightest possibility of accounting for it. In the meantime no pressure may have taken place, no tight shoe worn, no exposure to vicissitudes of heat or cold—nothing, in fact, that can throw the least light upon the subject; but to the surprise of the sufferer a corn upon whose disappearance he had congratulated himself, will not only be visible, but it will resist more than the ordinary means for its extirpation, and prove to be infinitely more obstinate than he could have imagined. Prompt attention is always demanded for those corns which are either dark in the centre or have any unusual colour, and more especially if these appearances are exhibited on the first approach of the enemy. They betoken that not only are the integuments in an unnatural state, but that the vascular and nervous system partakes of some unusual condition. I have uniformly observed that such cases neglected have been the most difficult I have had to encounter, and that I have had more uneasiness for the sake of my patient than I could willingly submit to. I also uniformly have found that corns between the toes have been very troublesome, and that the long interval of absence from pain is not to lead to the idea that they are becoming inert, and that they will remain so, for, sooner or later, to the great distress of the person who has to bear it, they will exhibit their real character. Pain, swelling, fever, misery of no ordinary description will arise, and will be difficult to subdue, without greater attention than can under ordinary cirumstances be paid. These are points which the superficial observer may be likely to overlook, but which I am convinced will be found of no small importance. If the patients who have corns did but know that they were their own enemies by their neglect of having recourse to proper assistance, less serious cases would present themselves, and half the occupation of the Chiropodist would be lost; still I feel it my duty to impress upon the minds of all "tuto, cito," if it were done, would that it were done quickly. All these things demand promptitude, and that must depend upon the determination of the sufferer to seek assistance as early as possible. The most remarkable cases which I have seen, would have been in their earlier stage of easy treatment, but either neglect or a want of judgment has rendered them difficult, and have demanded the most sedulous care. If then I have been so urgent upon these points, I must fall back upon the experience which has taught me the necessity of prompt and active measures to make up for the slowness, the indolence, or the inattention of those whose duty it was to have gone before me, and have rendered my interference altogether unnecessary.

There is no one who does not think himself equal to give advice upon medical subjects. An invalid always has a vast variety of friends who have something or other to recommend which they believe to be infallible, and as for corns, each person has his own undoubted plan. I lately read with much pleasure a work addressed to sportsmen, by Lieutenant-Colonel Hawker, entitled 'Instruction to Young Sportsmen in all that relates to Guns and Shooting.' He does not, however, confine himself to the mere description of the destructive instruments, but gives various pieces of advice. Amongst these is one from which I must most decidedly dissent, although his work may be valuable to others, and his instructions generally admired; as this opinion is not unfrequently entertained, I have given the extract with a view of recommending sufferers to avoid it.

"To walk with corns, and without torture, "get a piece of chamois leather, spread with "diachylon plaster. Cut with your wadding-"punch as many rounds as will form a sufficient "thickness to prevent the boot or shoe from "pressing your stocking on the corn; for the "reception of which you must punch a small "hole through the centre. By this simple con-

" trivance I have known many a dot-and-go-one " gentleman start off as bold as a dog just un- " coupled.

" The following recipe was given me by the " Earl of ——— on purpose for this book; and " I set my man to try it on several unfortunates " who have given him their blessing for the cures " he has made.

" Mercurial plaster - -	}	2 drachms of each.
" Diachylon ditto, with resin		
" Diachylon ditto - -		
" Sugar of lead - -		20 grains.

" All mixed together
" And spread on leather.

" Apply a piece of this plaster for three or " four days. Then soak the foot; and rub the " corn with a piece of pumice-stone. Again " repeat the plaster; and the corn will soon dis- " appear.—N.B. The corn never to be cut."

So far from being serviceable, although the relief is temporary, and, as the author observes, a gentleman may start off with apparent ease, yet upon that very spot soon grows an extraneous lump corresponding to the hole formed in the plaster; this is exceedingly difficult to get rid of, and becomes painful in the extreme, the circulation of the blood is checked by the surrounding leather, and the nerve painfully pressed on. Even when the corn is extracted this lump remains, so that the wearer of the plaster becomes subject all his life to a very distressing malady. Let me therefore recommend no chamois leather spread with diachylon with a hole in the centre for the reception of the corns—too late will the wearer find out the disadvantage of not attending to my counsel.

That corns have disappeared where diseases of an aggravated character have supervened is a matter of little doubt, and attempts have been made to explain the causes of this apparently singular circumstance, but the probability is that in the instances where this has occurred there has been in the first instance absolute repose of the whole body—there has been confinement to bed, no pressure whatever on any portion of the limbs, and at the same time much medicine has been taken, which removes the inflammatory condition of the body, and relieves any congestion of the vascular system. The nausea of sea sickness often produces a complete emptying out of the capillary vessels, and hence some of those cures which have been said to be effected by a sea voyage, but which after all are in many instances apocryphal. After a protracted fit of the gout it has often happened that for a time the most annoying corns have vanished, and the invalid has indulged in the fancy that the greater evil has driven away the lesser. These hopes are destined to meet with disappointment, for before many weeks have elapsed he has sensible demonstration that there was but a cessation of hostilities, for his enemy again invades his foot, and very probably takes up the precise position from which he was supposed to be driven; at other times there is a curious metastasis, the great toe has ceased to be the spot, and the little toe exhibits the malady in all its most striking features. The way in which the corn has been exfoliated is sufficiently marked to show that the nutrition has been cut off, for there is a large foramen; this, however, does not long exist. Cellular tissue is formed, or else again does the rete mucosum furnish its fluid to cause fresh depositions of the layers which constitute the principal portion of the corn. The same falling out of the corn has been known to follow several of the inflammatory and the exanthematous diseases. After variola or small-pox there has been sometimes a perfect cure; the pustular action having, it would appear, superseded the former abnormal state. This has likewise been the case after scarlet fever, and upon the production of a completely new epidermis there has been a total cessation of all excrescences on the feet. On the other hand they have been increased by the development of particular diseases, more especially those which affect the kidnies or the urinary secretion. There is such a sympathy existing between the organs which excrete the fluid and the skin, that we are not at a loss to account for diseases springing up in the one tissue where the other has had its usual condition altered, or where some of those changes which modern chemistry has so clearly shown have occurred. We cannot be surprised that after fractures of the limb, after any affection requiring for any length of time the horizontal position, that benefit has been derived. The altered state of the circulation, independent of the state of absolute quiescence, is sufficient to account for this; but it would be well could we be assured that there would be no recurrence. Such, however, is not the case; indeed, we never can be sufficiently on our guard, even under circumstances the most advantageous, against their re-appearance, notwithstanding the precautions that may be taken, unless they be founded upon proper principles. A change of climate has doubtless some influence. We find in the north people exceedingly subject to corns, whilst in warmer latitude they are scarcely to be found; then we must remember that, independent of the exceeding cold, the inhabitants are apt to wear very thick goloshes of an unyielding material over their shoes. In St Petersburg and in Stockholm Chiropodists are in great demand, and if thoroughly conversant with their duties would make large fortunes, besides holding a proper position in society. In the North of Germany corns are frequent, whilst in Rome, in Naples, or in Madrid they are not altogether so frequent; it is true that many of the social habits prevent this. Probably the female inhabitants of Castile have the most perfectly formed foot and ankle of any race of women, and corns are almost entirely unknown to them.

When we reflect how much the well-being of individuals depends upon domestic comfort and the attention to minute points which escape the notice of superficial observers, I feel persuaded that I shall not be supposed to have treated the subject of corns with more earnestness or with a greater degree of anxiety than is necessary, and that the long experience I have had fully justifies my attempt to impress upon the minds of those to whom the guardianship of infancy and of youth belongs, the absolute necessity of watchfulness. Studying as I have done under the first authorities, I have had my theories corrected and my opinions confirmed by practice.

CHAPTER III.

THE bunnion differs from the corn in the actual seat of the disease, for it involves the integuments generally, and is attended with active inflammation, so that the usual accompaniments of heat, swelling, and redness are attendant upon its progress. It is not to be considered as a simple induration of the mucus of the rete accompanied by a morbid state of the epidermis, but as an increase of the integuments which belong to the great toe. It has been confounded with corns and callosities, from a want of investigation into the actual nature of the disease. It runs the course of inflammation, and is liable to the various terminations which attend upon that state, for where resolution does not occur, there may be either effusion, suppuration, or mortification, though fortunately the instances are rare in which the worst form of the disease appears. The first phalanx of the toe has been so swollen, has put on such inflammatory action, that gout has been pronounced to be present where this enlargement has existed; and as those who are somewhat in the vale of years are more prone to be attacked by the annoyance, it has often led to the suspicion that it is in some measure connected with a gouty diathesis; the ordinary termination, however, of the affection, where it has been judiciously treated, so essentially differs from that of the constitutional disorder, that the mistake is easily rectified. The epidermis in such cases peels off in scales, such as are produced in the onion, from whence indeed it is supposed to derive its name, at any rate the similarity to the French word 'oignon,' would lead to such a conclusion. The bunnion must undoubtedly be admitted to be the result of pressure in the first instance, and is not unfrequently attended with a crop of corns, but it is essentially a different disease from the corn, and approaches more to the nature of the diseases which affect the articulation of the joints, involving many structures, and occasionally leaving behind it serious mischief; and although there may be temporary alleviation of the inflammatory symptoms, they are likely to recur, and often exhibit peculiar phenomena, which lead to the idea that there is some connexion with constitutional malady.

It certainly has often occurred that the bunnion has been mistaken for constitutional disease. We have known an eminent statesman upon whom a physician, who had distinguished himself by writing a large octavo on the gout, was in constant attendance, giving without remorse or dread, huge doses of colchicum and magnesia, and prescribing with great talent and skill all the usual well-accustomed draughts and mixtures which that ferocious enemy to the comforts of the great, the gout, usually demands. Upon his altar had been offered up innumerable gifts of phials and pill-boxes; still the enemy would maintain his position, nor leave the comfortable quarters in which the learned physician supposed he had installed himself, for some considerable length of time. The patient having been for some time affected with corns thought the present moment of repose a favourable one for the cure of these additional plagues. I was honoured with a summons; my first inspection convinced me that the "causa teterrima" in this instance was a well-marked bunnion. I felt it my duty, before offering my opinion myself on the subject, to seek an interview with the physician. It was graciously accorded to me, and upon my expressing what had struck me, he with great candour acknowledged that he had not seen the supposed gouty foot, for knowing how subject his patient was to its paroxysms, he had imagined that an incipient attack was the cause of his suffering. I was left by him to follow my own treatment after he was convinced that there was much of truth in my view of the case, for ocular inspection proved to him the enlargement of the integuments covering the first joint of the great toe, and that the cuticle was already thickened, and lay scaling, the whole foot partook of the irritation, and some febrile symptoms gave countenance to the idea entertained by the physician of the nature of the disease. A few hours were sufficient to restore to his usual state this gentleman. All that it was necessary for me to do was to apply a cataplasm of the simplest kind, and to enjoin a horizontal position. I was able a short time afterwards to give permanent relief, and obtained some little share of confidence for the manner in which I had acted, as well from the physician as from the patient, who remained perfectly ignorant that he had been treated for an attack to which he had not been subject. Similar cases have presented themselves to me in which I have had occasion to find medical men not so accurate in their diagnosis as they should be, from the carelessness with which they have been accustomed to treat the diseases of the feet. They have been taught to look down upon them as trifles altogether beneath their consideration, the consequence of which has been that they have mistaken diseases which demanded the simplest treatment, for others which must be actively met, or the system will succumb. It is true, since Sir Benjamin Brodie has in his masterly treatise explained some of the phenomena attendant upon disease of the joints, that more just estimates have been formed of the nature of those affections to which the numerous joints of the foot are subject, and the real cause of some of the diseases more precisely ascertained.

The treatment of the bunnion, above all the maladies to which the integuments of the foot are liable, must depend upon the general skill and well-founded experience of the practitioner. The eye and tact are absolutely requisite to decide upon what class of remedies he is to depend. Cold applications, warm fomentations, are to be employed, not indiscriminately, but according to the actual appearances which are developed. The remedies which in one instance are highly beneficial, may be detrimental in another; and it is only from the actual ocular inspection of the state of the foot that we can give directions as to the course to be pursued. It is one of those instances which the opposers of nosological systems have so often brought forward. You call certain symptoms by a certain name, and you then have recourse to a certain class of remedies, which have been found to be efficacious in that disease, forgetting that in each individual instance there are symptoms peculiar to it. You may call an aggregate number of symptoms the gout, and you may then immediately prescribe colchicum; but the wise practitioner knows that colchicum is not good in every stage of the gout; and that there are certain circumstances under which it is not advantageously given. Thus it is with the malady of which I have been speaking. When a bunnion is present, the best application, says a popular author, is an application of a cataplasm of oatmeal and ground linseed, renewed twice a day; this appears in a volume which was formerly in the hands of almost all who were interested in the subjects of our discussion; it was the hand-book to which most men referred, the guide whose authority was sufficient for all; but serious would be the consequences if every bunnion was thus indiscriminately treated; suppuration and the worst consequences would ensue, and though we are told that should purulent matter be formed, we have nothing to do but to keep the abscess clean and not irritate it, those who have had to treat such abscesses, and still more those who have had to encounter them, know what time is consumed, what pain is borne, and what irritation arises from such an occurrence. This plan may well be followed where resolution by other means cannot be prevented; the inflammation must, if possible, be speedily brought to resolution; the cold spirituous lotion, mindererus' spirit, goulard solutions, are in general first to be had recourse to; but sometimes, and here is judgment absolutely necessary, warm decoction of poppies, infusion of camomile flowers, cataplasms of various kinds are the proper remedies. Indeed I will scarcely venture to lay down decisive rules, for everything must vary according to circumstances. The nitro-muriatic pediluvium, the mustard pediluvium, the acetous, all are capable of affording relief. The most judicious plan is to be guided by symptoms, to do nothing that can keep up irritation, to soothe and palliate rather than attempt to drive away by active means a malady which may, by injudicious treatment, become a source of much pain and lasting annoyance. I most earnestly recommend that leeches should not be employed; the quantity drawn by them is never sufficient to do any good, and much time is lost which might be advantageously employed by other means. This plan, which is followed upon every occasion where inflammation occurs by surgeons in England, often is attended with mischievous effects, and leaves behind a degree of debility sometimes difficult to be overcome. How often have I known a sufferer, first tormented with leeches, with hot poultices, and then caustic, who would have been quickly cured by simpler means, and would have avoided, probably, a long confinement. I would impress upon the minds of those who are afflicted with bunnions that they never can be thoroughly cured until every vestige of the stem or root is skilfully removed. If careful instruction be given, the enlargement of the joint will thoroughly disappear.

I have just observed that there is something so resembling the appearance of a fit of the gout where a bunnion is present, that a skilful physician has been misled. Indeed, if attention be not paid to the state of the constitution, this may occur without much difficulty, for the tumefaction, pain, and redness, which attend upon both, require the experienced eye to detect which of the two it is. Before an examination of the foot it is always necessary to hear the statement of the patient, and you may most generally form an accurate diagnosis from the detail of his symptoms; for, although there may be constitutional derangements attendant upon the bunnion, as well as upon gout, yet I have always observed them to be of a different character. The gout is ushered in by a train of symptoms peculiar to itself—the flatulence, heart-burn, and the dyspeptic signs are of a very marked character, more especially in those who once have had a paroxysm. The febrile state, too, is one of a high degree of irritation, of which the mind partakes as well as the body. From bunnion there is an excruciating pain during the night, but there is not that singular sensation which has been so admirably described by Sydenham, of utter impossibility of finding a position that is a relief from pain. That great physician was himself a martyr to the gout, and if he had during the paroxysm minuted down each varying sensation as it arose, he could not more accurately have described this disease as it presents itself under ordinary circumstances, and in the greater number of cases in which it affects individuals. The pain supervenes in bunnion sometime after the swelling, whilst in gout the violent lancinating pain comes on before there is any appearance whatever of inflammatory symptoms about the part where the disease is to show itself; the pain, too, generally confines itself to the joint of the toe—the foot, and the ankle do not sympathise, as is the case in gout; the paroxysm of this latter disease commonly commences early in the morning and remits towards evening, whilst the bunnion is generally relieved after the night's sleep, and it is in consequence of the fatigue of the day that it shows itself in its worst character towards evening. There is seldom that exquisite sensibility to the touch which makes the gouty person dread the approach of any one to him. By this explanation the reader will have some knowledge of the means by which the two affections should be distinguished, even without ocular demonstration.

CHAPTER IV.

THE callosity differs from the corn in the actual seat of the disease; it is the epidermis, which becomes thickened, and most frequently in considerable masses, when great pressure has for any length of time existed. The structure of the epidermis does not appear to be changed, as in the corn, for the external aspect of the integument remains much as it did in its previous state. Some callosities are remarkable for the extent over which they spread, occupying not unfrequently the largest portion of the sole of the foot; and frequently there is one on the joint immediately beneath the little toe. This callosity is often interspersed with many little spots or corns; this gives considerable pain, and has the appearance of a large protuberance, something similar to the bunnion, which occupies only the large toe; indeed, some inexperienced persons have made this mistake, but it is right that I should correct a misstatement made by so many authors, that more than one bunnion has appeared on each foot at a time; this cannot be the case, for it is only the joint of the great toe which is subject to this disease. Sometimes there is scarcely any swelling, but pain and heat are felt on the joint of the great toe, where in a little time there will be found a bunnion, which always occupies that part of the foot, and never exists elsewhere, so that it is impossible there could be two bunnions on one foot. This is the callosity which must have been misnamed a bunnion. There are, however, cases in which, like a corn, it is limited to a small spot, and then there is some slight difficulty in the diagnosis, at least by those who have not enjoyed the practical opportunity of becoming familiar with all the varieties of the defects which present themselves in the feet where there is any deviation from the ordinary laws of nature. Sometimes a corn will shoot up in the very centre of the indurated mass, arising most probably from the irritation produced upon the rete mucosum. There are few persons who are entirely free from some callosity; occasionally they pass altogether unnoticed. They give neither annoyance nor pain; they remain stationary, neither enlarging nor diminishing, but furnishing an additional protection to an otherwise tender and easily acted-on surface. It not unfrequently occurs that, although during a very long period a callosity has never been the source of the slightest uneasiness, it, from some unexplained cause, or more probably from an alteration in the sort of boot or shoe worn, suddenly exhibits its power of diminishing the comforts of life; first, a sense of heat, of tingling, of shooting, is perceptible, and gradually inconvenience, annoyance, and even severe pain are felt. And, under such circumstances, I find that it is generally believed that there is more difficulty in effecting a cure than where it had been perceived at an early stage, and had met with that attention which every disordered state requires; but my own experience tells me that however late the sufferer seeks relief, that it may be given if the plan I propose be followed. The edges of the heels, the outer ball of the great toe, the soles of the feet, and various parts of the surface of the little toes, are more or less the objects of the invasion of these disagreeable callosities. They bear a considerable resemblance, both in the proximate and exciting causes, to those indurations of the dermoid coverings which occur in the hands, on the shoulders, the knees, and the elbows of persons occupied in various of the departments of life, in which pressure upon these portions of the body takes place, and more especially if any degree of friction accompanies the pressure. The knees of women employed in scouring or cleaning exhibit something of this kind, whilst the hardness of the integuments of the palms of the hands of those occupied in the manipulation demanded in mechanics may also be justly compared with that which is found on various parts of the feet.

Looking at the callosity in its worst state—examining all the circumstances which are connected with it, and the numerous examples which have fallen under my superintendence—I should say that to the experienced man there is no great difficulty, but to the uninitiated there is a great deal, which I hope I shall be enabled to show him is to be avoided. On dissecting away the integument there will be found numerous stems embedded in cells which bear every resemblance to the ordinary corn; these must altogether be thoroughly, completely, and carefully removed. They must be eradicated by gentle, but certain means; they are not to be cut out, but taken away by an instrument properly formed, and it must be borne in mind that if they are not all removed there will be the probability, nay, even the certainty of a return. The great skill of the Chiropodist is here exhibited; he is not to perform a showy operation, but he is to extirpate, by gradual but certain manipulation, that which is at present troublesome, and would, if any small portion be allowed to remain, become a cause of future sorrow. I would impress upon the minds of those who may have such cases that they are not to be misled by the apparent facility with which they can operate, for wounds here are most dangerous. We have to dread, where ignorance and rashness are too predominant, convulsions, lock-jaw, and those sad terminations which I have already alluded to.

There is a circumstance which is particularly remarkable with regard to these callosities, which is, that they are not, like corns, the effect of the pressure produced in walking, or by tight shoes, which undoubtedly must be considered the usual exciting cause of these annoyances, for they are found to occur with great frequency amongst those who take little pedestrian exercise, who wear the easiest shoes, and who are particularly sedentary. It is a curious fact that those who ride on horse-back and are amongst the foremost in the chase, are strikingly liable to these affections. We have known men who are remarkable for their love of hunting, who have no other rural pursuit to which they are partial, who neither shoot nor fish, and who, when in town, take little but carriage exercise, suffer in a singular degree from hard, thickened, callous indurations around the heel, and they are not unfrequently exceedingly sensitive. The whole epidermis is in such cases unusually dry, ragged, and small papulæ in groups cover its surface ; those who are advanced in years seem to be more subject to the rapid advance of these indurations, and they seldom can check them unless they have frequent recourse to the pediluvium of a high temperature, followed by rubbing the surface for some considerable length of time with a rough dry towel; indeed many persons have found their only relief from following this plan systematically for a considerable length of time, and even if they have abandoned it, from the total absence of the callosity, they have found it to return and to become even more troublesome than before. It does sometimes happen that nature herself performs a cure, and the disorganized substance falls off, or is rubbed off, and this is now and then done as effectually and as clearly as it would be by the knife, or by arsenic applied to a cancerous or schirrous surface; but a large foramen is usually left, which sometimes for a considerable length of time exists without being filled up; at others an unusual growth appears with several corns in the centre; there are indeed numerous varieties of these callosities, which experience can alone attempt to describe, explain, or cure. There is one, however, which I cannot pass by in silence, because when it does occur it puts the patient to the greatest inconvenience and suffering. It is when the induration takes place on the apex of the great toe immediately in the skin in contact with the nail. Its commencement is so insensible and gradual that it is not unusual that it entirely escapes observation until it begins to assume a serious character and to be accompanied with tumefaction, heat, redness, and pain. A thin superficies of the skin is at first the only seat of callus, and this induration is probably unnoticed until the whole of the immediate neighbourhood is involved in the same state; the skin becomes almost transparent, the nail partakes of the diseased action, its root adds to the irritation, the pain is often so acute as to prevent sleep, the constitution, probably naturally irritable, is more or less influenced by it; of course all attempt at movement is quite out of the question, for its consequence would, independent of the pain produced, be most serious. This callus is not large, but most probably, from its embracing much of the nervous papillæ that are distributed over the toes, becomes the source of all those inconveniences just mentioned, and which, when I have been called upon to remedy, I have found to produce serious effect upon the health.

CHAPTER V.

WARTS have found more distinguished surgical inquirers than corns; the frequency of their occurrence on the hands, and the unsightly appearance which they there present, have most probably led to the investigations which even John Hunter did not disdain to pursue; but after all that has been done, and after even microscopic examination, the exact nature of these "plague spots," as they have been termed by one who was infested with them, and could by no means suggested to him entirely eradicate them, is not understood. Various, however, have been the attempts to ascertain from what particular portion of the dermoid coverings they spring, and the contradictory opinions only serve to show how unequal is the best judgment of a single individual upon some of apparently the most trivial of the works of nature. Some of the various forms in which these excrescences appear evidently show that they are in some measure connected with the constitution; and though they wear the form of a local disorder, yet are they more or less influenced by some state of health which is not fully understood. The wart differs from the corn in its texture; more organized matter enters into its composition, as is evinced by the facility with which bleeding is produced when the slightest incision has been made; nor is it so thick, hard, horny, or impenetrable, although it has a surface occasionally of much roughness, hardness, and thickness. Their attachment to the body is altogether of a different character — they burrow more completely under the surface of the integument, and are held on by a species of peduncle sometimes of great broadness; at others, of very slight and pendulous form. To describe them would be out of the question, for their general characters are well known; they seem, however, in modern days to be much less frequent, even among schoolboys, than they were. Whether this is attributable to greater cleanliness, or to different habits of life, I will not attempt to discuss; but certain it is that the cases are rarer than they were, and even in large schools they do not infest the hands of boys with the same inveteracy they did formerly. They do occasionally occur, and sometimes attain a considerable size, when there would seem to be no means of accounting for their origin or development. Improper nutrition has been said to be one of the frequent sources of these excrescences; rye bread, and beans (substituted, when roasted, for coffee), have had these deformities laid to their charge;

others, again, have spoken of the secretion of the kidneys being surcharged with acid, which, not carried away, has been borne into the small cuticular papillæ, which have become enlarged. Nor have some theorists been wanting in what has been called extravagance, who have assigned to globules of mercury taken by the parents the "fons et origo malorum." It has been said that they are pustules containing an infinitesimal portion of some other of the mineral or organic bodies which have not found their due action in nature's laboratory, the stomach, and are therefore to be elsewhere expelled by the "vis medicatrix naturæ."

The humoral pathologists have been more than usually eloquent upon these apparently little foes to health, and have talked of the expulsion of gross morbific matter unfortunately stopped in its career, and determined to the surface of the skin, where, not meeting with a proper mode of escape, it has caused inflammation of the papillæ, subsequent formation of callosity, and consequent alteration of structure. As it is not for me, "tantas conponere lites," I will not further discuss the matters connected with their origin than to say that they appear to be a congeries of vessels surrounded by a thin coating of epidermis, the rete mucosum, and the cutis vera.

It might indeed be a subject of medical inquiry, not unworthy the highest of those intellectual men who devote themselves to the relief of their fellow beings, what is the precise nature of these diseased portions of the skin; for there are many circumstances which lead to a belief that they are more intimately blended with the constitution than we are at first sight led to allow, for often they seem indications of specific diseases. They are found to accompany some of those loathsome affections to which human nature is prone, and they are also found in some instances to wear a remarkable cancerous tendency, running, after long existence in a quiescent state, into active disease ; we find, too, that when they occur in large numbers upon various parts of the body, and return again with great quickness, after they have apparently been eradicated, that they more or less affect the whole of the system, and that elderly people are not so subject to them as the young and active ; that when they do make their appearance they are not apt to remain in an indolent state, but to put on a degree of active inflammation, which demands the most serious attention. The point connected with contagion is one of curious, but at present of unsatisfactory inquiry ; for although from cases beyond suspicion it has been seen that an infected person has conveyed them to another, yet, on the other hand, so many other instances exist where there has not been the slightest contamination, although every facility has existed, and even inoculation has failed, that many persons altogether deny its possibility. It may, however, be affirmed, as I believe may be said of almost all contagious and infectious disorders, that where there is a predisposition in an individual to a particular complaint, the slightest exposure will prove sufficient for his imbibing it; and, on the other hand, some individuals are altogether incapable of being in the slightest degree affected, even when exposed to the virulence in its most concentrated form. The pain which results from these excrescences is generally very trifling, unless they are of a large size, are in a bad position, or have put on any strikingly diseased action; and they may exist for a considerable length of time on the hands without producing any uneasiness whatever. Upon the feet, however, they are much more likely to become speedily a source of much annoyance, and sometimes they have been known from untoward circumstances to become a matter of much moment. I have seen indeed cases in which maladies of a much more dangerous kind have been borne with greater fortitude and philosophy than when warts have at first been the only complaint. It is when they have been seated on the sole of the foot, or upon the toes, that they have worn a form likely to produce considerable mischief, and to be the cause of pain of the most excruciating kind. It can well be understood how in such situations they are kept in a state of miserable irritation, every movement of the body operating upon them, and keeping them in a state of constant inflammation. The slightest touch aggravates them; they are incessantly exposed to friction, to pressure, to bruises, they are pinched, squeezed, tormented, until at last ulcers of a very serious nature are produced, and then commences a long train of acute suffering and of insupportable agony, such as those only who have endured or seen others afflicted by, can form the slightest conception. A more ingenious method of torture could not have been found for the regicide Damian, nor for the miserable martyrs who fell into the clutches of the holy Inquisition.

This may appear an exaggerated picture, but I have known such cases where, too, corns have been supposed to be present. A case occurred to me in Cork during a short visit. Dr William Murphy, an eminent physician in extensive practice there, had long suffered from a wart on the sole of his foot, which he fancied a corn. He had been under the care of persons who professed themselves capable of relieving him. He placed himself under my care, a single operation cured him; and some years have elapsed without the recurrence of a single inconvenience. He, previously to my examination, told me that he would with pleasure confine himself for four or five days if necessary, and was as much pleased as he was surprised to find immediately after the operation that he was perfectly capable of following his occupations in a much easier manner than he had been enabled to do for a long time. All that is demanded on such occasions is a thorough knowledge of what can be done. I have no secret, I have no nostrum; experience and attention are what I rely upon.

A curious chapter might be written upon the popular ideas which have existed with regard to warts and the means which have been adopted for their cure. It would illustrate the history of the progress of true science—it would show how ignorance is led by pretended wisdom, how often superstition and the dread of some unknown agency will induce persons to try as remedies the most extraordinary substances, and to place a firm belief in supernatural assistance. That those who feel only astonishment at the mysteries of

Nature, without any attempt to ascertain on what they depend, should blindly rush forward and grasp at any object recommended to them for the relief of their ailments, cannot so much surprise us, but we cannot withhold our astonishment and regret when we find men capable of penetrating a portion of the veil which hides from the world at large the region of truth fondly and foolishly placing their faith in inert substances, and having recourse to charms, to spells, and to various absurdities, when they might much more easily look for truer and for better things. In the list of medical authorities who have fostered popular prejudices, and perhaps have earnestly believed in the truth of their mysterious remedies, we find names of great eminence—men who have distinguished themselves not only as the collectors together of the experience of others, but who themselves have possessed both the power and the wish to investigate the value of medicinal substances. Boerhaave and Sauvages were not free from these faults, and there are many who have collected together the instances of credulity. Can it be really believed that a professor in a university of some reputation would instil upon the minds of his patients the doctrine that the lichens which are said to be found upon the dead body of a murdered person can effectually cure warts; or that another philosopher equally eminent should assert that from his own experience they were to be completely eradicated by means of a thread extracted from the linen near the arm-pit of a person executed for crime; that another should prescribe the stealing of a small piece of the sirloin of beef from a butcher's shop, burying it beneath the ground, and believe that as it slowly disorganized so would the warts decay. A few words muttered over the disordered part were affirmed to be completely efficacious, if the person who pronounced them was the seventh son of a seventh son. The fasting saliva has long been held as a decided cure, as also the mucus issuing from the snail, the bezoar, the rubbing daily with a diamond, and many other sagacious ideas have issued from men's minds, and their believers have been tempted to follow the advice; and as not unfrequently these warts disappear without any adequate reason, their departure is ascribed to the wondrous power of the favourite remedy, and "post hoc, propter hoc" is a quite sufficient ground for further trial of the important agent. There is little doubt that many of the families of particular classes in the vegetable kingdom act upon warts—some of them by their acrid powers, others by their natural acids. In the class Ranunculaceæ we find several families and their species which evidently possess considerable powers of action upon the integuments of the skin, and have been employed both popularly and scientifically for some length of time with considerable success, but they are not all of them entirely innocuous. One or two species of the genus ranunculus have a very curative juice, whilst if some others are mistaken for it they produce considerable mischief. The ranunculus acris possesses very striking properties, and has been used with much success, but the sceleratus has been known, when employed, to blister the skin in a most striking manner, producing considerable ulceration, attended with an effusion of a very acrid lymph, which, burrowing in the surrounding cellular membrane, has caused very extensive tumefaction, attended with numbness, and sensation of torpor throughout the whole of the upper extremity. There are others of this genus which are equally productive of annoyance. In this order stands the delphinium stavisagria, a herb which certainly deserves the favourable notice which it gained from our older herbalists; the part of the plant employed is the powder of the root; this sprinkled over a wart acts as a mild escharotic, seldom producing any irritation, and under its employments occasionally the largest warts have disappeared; and it is a well-ascertained fact, that when warts of considerable magnitude disappear, all the smaller ones in its immediate neighbourhood follow so good an example. The skin seems to undergo a change, and new action throughout the surface of the surrounding parts seems to be rapidly put on. Amongst the umbelliferous class are found several families which are actually to be depended upon in the very early stage of warts, before they have acquired any large size, or become prominent—the conium maculatum, the æthusa cynapium, the cuminum cyminum; the latter is a very favourite remedy in many parts of Europe, for the resolution of affections of the skin, for scrofulous enlargements or tumors;

the seeds applied in little bags, rendered warm, have considerable influence. This is the plant which the Romans extol so highly, for its effects as a detergent, and certainly when taken internally it has much power over the whole surface of the skin, although it seems to have no remedial agency in actual diseases of the coverings; it drives away blotches, maculæ, warts, and excrescences which disfigure. Dioscorides, and Galen more especially, allude to its power upon the face, whilst Avicenna recommends its external use to beautify the complexion; this it is that the student took when he wished to appear in Rome as the deep-reading man; the disciples of the Orator Porcius Latro, who desired to imitate their master in the delicate paleness of his countenance, as well as in his oratory, were in the habit of drinking of the "pallentis grana cumini." Several other herbs might be enumerated, many of which doubtless have gained celebrity from the friction which has been employed; for sometimes, when accident has caused the surrounding part to be inflamed, the absorbents have quickly carried away the heterogeneous mass which has incumbered it. What have I to say of the spider's cobweb, were I to give my sanction in its favour, might I not be ranked amongst those whom I have just noticed, not only as credulous themselves, but as the cause of credulity in others; but I have certainly heard some narratives, although I have no experience myself, which would stagger my disbelief. It has been said that this animal secretion has slight caustic power; that it arrests bleeding from small vessels there can be no doubt, but that may arise from its producing a coagulum, which many thin substances, such as cotton, thread, or fur, will do.

After all, however, that has been written, and well weighing the numerous recipes that exist, I firmly believe that there are but two ways of altogether getting rid of these troublesome disfigurements; the one, by dispersing and acting upon them by means of corroding or caustic substances; the other, under certain circumstances, by excision. These are the only means by which we can altogether assure ourselves of success; for they may last for a considerable length of time whilst inefficient treatment is followed, and they may give rise to a crop of similar substances on some other portion of the hands. The actual cautery, or the burning off warts, has very properly been long since abandoned, for it was found that only the external surface was acted upon; in some instances, however, a red-hot wire passed through the body of the wart has been speedily followed by its total disappearance. The hydrochlorate of ammonia dissolved in water, and the hydrochlorate of lime are the most certain means of destroying them; the process, however, in both instances is very slow, and demands perseverance, for if discontinued before the proper time, no advantage is derived. The warts are to be kept constantly moist with the solution of one or other of these neutral salts, small folds of linen are to be soaked in it, and applied at night; but this must be duly attended to. It must not be the practice for two or three days, and then laid aside; it must be followed up for a month, at the end of which time it will be found that the excrescence no longer exists, and it will not again return. Success almost always follows upon this plan, and therefore it is the one I would urge as that upon which the greatest reliance can be placed. The most obstinate warts, that had baffled the attention of the most skilful, and that had re-appeared after other treatment, completely yielded to this; and since it has become under ordinary circumstances the plan I recommend to be pursued. Nitric acid, as a caustic remedy, has been extensively used, but it requires judgment and a careful application; it is not to be indiscriminately employed, it is not to be looked upon as a domestic remedy which may or may not be tried, according to the caprice of an individual. It is capable of being mischievous; those, therefore, who use it must have experience and reason to guide them. A drop upon the centre of the wart is all that is required; sometimes the diluted acid will succeed where the concentrated fails. Excision demands tact, is painful, and is not to be performed by the uninitiated. Much of the same dexterity which the corn requires must be shown for warts; and, although we need not apprehend danger, we must remember that there are many bad effects consequent upon ill-judged incision. Ligature by a thread, if there be a simple pendulous basis, will often be quite enough; if not, the caustic potash, or nitrate of silver, may be gently applied to the surface remaining. Warts on the soles of the feet are oftentimes most troublesome, and are to be treated with great tenderness, for they are sometimes irritable, and are accompanied by itching of an annoying character, and a species of tickling which is almost as insupportable as direct pain. The next object of my consideration must be to point out the means by which these diseases — whether they are of a trifling or an aggravated character — may be avoided; for it would not be productive of benefit to the reader or to the practitioner simply to state what is to be done when maladies are present, but to show what precautions may be taken to prevent their approach. The old adage, "Prevention is better than cure," is as judicious as it is necessary; and if we cannot, from the habits of life, pay quite as much attention to the feet as to the hands, we may, nevertheless, remember how much of good is to be derived from care. Although the feet are more out of immediate sight, they are still most important members of the individual.

CHAPTER VI.

THE management of the feet has been, in the preceding pages, the subject of a vast variety of hints from me, yet I think that, even with the accusation of a repetition of my recommendations, and the fear of being somewhat tedious, I may point out some circumstances which are essentially necessary to the comforts of life, and which may be considered of no small importance when we reflect that, as age advances, everything that tends to render us incapable of taking moderate exercise, that produces inconvenience, fatigue, and listlessness, must shorten the period of existence, and render those later days, which ought to be spent in cheerfulness and serenity, dwelling upon the past in order to prepare ourselves for the future, uncomfortable to bear. The greater the care of the minutiæ, or what are often termed the trifles of life, the less will there be of the peevishness and moroseness which too often accompany the end of our career; and few there are who, in the height of early joys, when "youth is at the prow, and pleasure at the helm," think that, however "fair laughs the morn," the bark will not always glide smoothly down the stream, and therefore carelessly listen to the admonition of those who have had experience. The young pedestrian, who, with knapsack on his back, scales the summits of the lofty Ben Lomond, or who perambulates, untired, the valleys of Switzerland, and congratulates himself that he can walk forty miles a day, might preserve his powers with little deterioration if, during these praiseworthy excursions, which ought to bring health and knowledge, he pays due attention to those humble instruments by whose means he attains so much enjoyment. By following a proper system not only may he traverse all parts of the world uninjured and in comfort, but he may be enabled to do so, though probably not with the same vigour, when the snow begins to appear on his head, and when generally activity and power of walking cease in individuals. By careful attention to his shoes, which should be large enough to admit of the natural swelling of the feet; by wearing stockings of soft and yielding material, which fit without leaving much margin either at the toes or at the heels; by carefully sponging the feet at the end of the day's progress with cold water impregnated with salt; and by gentle friction with a hard towel, keeping the legs for a short time after exercise in a relaxed position—he will be ready for the next day's march without feeling lassitude or inconvenience. Should the least blister appear, it must be opened with a needle, the foot kept immersed in warm water until every portion of the effused fluid is discharged; this is assisted by gentle pressure, and friction must for a short time afterwards be persevered in.

It is almost a work of supererogation for me to point out the absolute necessity of foot cleanliness to a civilized and cultivated people; every one who has the slightest self-respect or desire for health must be too well aware of the necessity of constant ablution; holy writ has proclaimed that "cleanliness is next to godliness," and though probably it may be rather intended for the heart and for the intellect, yet as a moral duty it cannot be too frequently inculcated. One of the greatest duties, both according to the Mosaic dispensation, and also the commands of the Mahometan lawgiver, is frequent ablution. I have always found that this duty is best attended to, if it is followed with determined regularity; two evenings in the week the feet should be immersed in the warm pediluvium, about ninety degrees of Fahrenheit is a temperature that is generally preferable, somewhat higher is required for persons more advanced in life, but above one hundred degrees is seldom desirable; besides this, morning and evening, careful sponging with either hot or cold water should be attended to. In early life the habit of plunging the feet into cold water, morning and evening, may be fairly and properly inculcated; but this must not be commenced at a late period of life; more especially the cold water at night should be avoided, for apoplexy, gout in the stomach, and other diseases may supervene upon injudiciously commencing such new practices. Sir Astley Cooper, than whom no man ever enjoyed better health, and who lived to a later period than the ordinary days of life, used to state in those valuable lectures which for a series of years he delivered for the benefit of medical science, that he attributed his well-being to his daily immersing his feet in cold water as soon as he arose, and to his use of a rough towel immediately after it. In the coldest day of winter he was to be seen without a great coat, with silk stockings on his legs, and short breeches, traversing the court of the hospital, or sitting in his carriage. Numerous indeed are the instances in which this truly hydropathic cure for affections of the feet has been attended with signal success. Hot water is apt to make the feet tender and susceptible; hence it is that I do not recommend the heat to be above ninety degrees. If the water is above ninety-eight degrees, or what is generally termed blood heat, there is a tendency to an undue determination of the blood, and the vascular system becomes too full, besides which there is not unfrequently some degree of feverishness produced; as a remedial agent, however, the heat may be increased,—I now speak of it merely as necessary for personal cleanliness.

The sponge should be most sedulously applied to the ankle, between the toes, and around the nails — these are the portions which more absolutely demand strict watch, and they should be thoroughly dried by the towel, no part should remain at all moist or damp. There is no objection to using afterwards a little eau de Cologne, or aromatic vinegar, or the Mindererus' spirit. The evaporation which they occasion is cool and comfortable. It is not right to leave the feet, after this, long exposed to the action of the air; the stocking should be drawn quickly on, and a loose slipper worn for some little time. It is seldom right to keep the feet in cold air after immersion in hot water; this, however, depends upon the condition of the individual; those who are delicate must necessarily be more cautious than the robust, who are seldom affected by such inconsiderable circumstances. Those who suffer from immoderate perspiration of the feet should use a solution of the chlorate of lime or of soda for its prevention, more especially if it be attended by any fœtor, which sometimes occurs, but more generally as an indication of constitutional disorder than of local affection. The sponge, moistened with equal parts of camphor julep, of Mindererus' spirit, with a few drops of spirits of lavender, will often put a stop to the most disagreeable effluvium which arises. The frequent change of the stocking during a hot day is necessary to some persons —to all it is a luxury—but is scarcely needed. In thus giving advice for the preservation of the feet, it must be remembered that the active and the inactive are to be considered by me, and that I have laid down general rules for the guidance of all, but there are many circumstances which would naturally modify my treatment. I would have every one careful, whilst he is studying the precepts best adapted for his own case, to remember that there may be too much attention as well as too little; that too much delicacy is as injudicious as too much carelessness. The equilibrium of health is to be maintained by a knowledge of what is to be done, and by judiciously carrying into practice those rules which carry with them the semblance of truth; that it is impossible to lay down one unchangeable rule, as all men are not equally adapted to the bed of Procrustes, so neither are one set of regulations to be followed by all. Each person is marked with peculiarities; and, as no two faces are precisely similar, so are there no parts of the body in two individuals bearing precisely the same stamp, or obedient to the same influences; but there are general and defined laws which regulate all things, and enable us to arrive at conclusions which embrace the larger portion of that which has been created.

The time necessary for keeping the feet in warm water must be noticed by me, because it is not unfrequent for persons to entertain the idea that they should be immersed for a considerable length of time in order to be productive of the end required. This is a great mistake, all the benefit which is to be derived may be obtained in about ten minutes, and all further foot-bathing is not only useless, but may in some instances be prejudicial, leaving behind a sense of weariness, undue heat, and sometimes pulsation of the arteries. One great objection to the long employment of hot water, which has not been often pointed out, but which not unfrequently arises, is the production of what are termed varicose veins. The vascular system losing its due equilibrium, the result has been that tumid state of the veins which is often very difficult of remedy. Some persons are apt to keep the feet in the bath, and to go on adding hot water as the first quantity cools down: this is injudicious, for all that is required is to immerse them for the length of time I have pointed out. Bran is occasionally added to the water, sometimes the powder of mustard seed, and small quantities of acids; these, however, demand the consideration of the medical man; certain it is that the hydrochloric and the nitric acids may be made, through the pediluvium, to have considerable influence upon the general as well as the local state. During the summer the bathing should be more frequent than in the winter, if the habit of bathing twice a week, as I have recommended, be not pursued. After this, friction with a hard, dry towel should be strictly persevered in.

I am no advocate for the use of the flesh brush; I find there is not that hard rubbing which is necessary, and that, from the unevenness of the surface of the hairs, there is not that general effect produced; besides which, itching and much irritation not unfrequently follows upon this treatment. The great desideratum is to render the feet perfectly dry, taking care that the pores of the epidermis are kept quite free from any laminæ which impede the proper perspiration. Besides this usual immersion, the simple sponging with luke-warm water, morning and evening, will be productive of a high degree of comfort, and will promote that general and local ease which all who value thc blessings of a healthy state will be most anxious to enjoy.

What sort of stockings do you recommend? is a question very often put to me, and I must confess it is one that I sometimes feel that I cannot answer to the satisfaction of my patients, for I know such is the general and very deserved preference given to the silk stocking, that I shall not satisfy my inquirer by advising the use of any other. It is, however, fortunate that silk, which from its material is so flexible, and so ornamental, is from other causes the best; yet there are circumstances under which worsted or woollen may be far preferable. Were I to tell a delicate young lady, whose foot and ankle are the theme of admiration, and make her "the observed of all observers," that she would enjoy dancing most in woollen stockings, feel less fevered, and be infinitely less tired, with whatever respect I might be listened to, I know that I dare not anticipate obedience; as the fair Narcissa proclaimed "woollen odious," so do I feel that the same epithet would be applied to my advice in stockings. Yet how much better would a fair one feel on the following day. At the same time I do not consider, for the mere ordinary occupation of dancing, for the transient amusement of the time, that it is necessary to discard the silk stocking. I merely mean to say, that where much muscular movement occurs, where there is much perspiration, woollen is very advantageously worn, it is very far superior to cotton and linen; both these substances become, after a time, saturated with the moisture from the feet, are then hardened, will absorb no more, and generate lasting inconvenience. The soldier on a long day's march feels the difference between a stocking of worsted and of cotton. He knows that the former will enable him to bear twice the quantity of fatigue—that he will have less chance of blisters—that he has nothing hard, cold, and stiff between his foot and his shoe; and although the day be exceeding hot, and perspiration flow with unabated vigour, he feels that he derives the greater comfort from that which at first appears too hot, and too likely to superinduce fatigue. I have elsewhere spoken of silk as the best material for stockings, especially in the winter; and, under all circumstances, it is doubtless preferable. It is singular to find that the Parisian ladies, so fond of displaying the beauty of the foot and ankle, always give the preference to cotton stockings; they require the most delicate texture, and are of opinion that they are the most elegant. They, however, are generally great sufferers from affections of the feet, and there is more room for study of the deviations from the healthy state of the foot to be found in Paris than elsewhere; indeed there is a singular sensibility and nervous susceptibility about them, which may in some measure arise from the want of proper pavement in Paris, and the determination to have the smallest possible foot. Indeed, there are more candidates for Cinderella's pigmy slipper in that gay metropolis than in all the rest of Europe. Care should be taken that the stocking is not too short for the foot ; few there are who pay attention to this point. The toes become cramped, and this is often worse than shoes that pinch the feet ; more especially should this be attended to in early youth, when the full development is taking place. Many of the disfigurements which are attributed to inattention to the shoe arise from this cause.

CHAPTER VII.

THE nails are not subject to diseases of so serious a character as those which we have already described; yet a work upon the treatment of the feet would not be complete without a general inquiry into the circumstances immediately connected with them. They perform some important functions in the human economy; and though probably not of so much importance to man in the highly civilized state into which his exertions have brought him, still they are not to be passed over as unimportant. Doubtless, to tribes dependent entirely for their daily subsistence upon the means with which Nature has endowed them for their varied pursuits of hunting, of fishing, and of gathering from the earth the herbs which they require, a substance which is not unlike the claws of quadrupeds or the beaks of birds might be absolutely necessary. The more polished races of man look upon them rather as ornamental additions than as serviceable instruments in agriculture, or as means of warfare; certain it is that they are now of little use to us, though they may defend the utmost ends of the extremities against the vicissitudes of temperature, or diminish the intensity of the sense of touch. The nails naturally divide themselves into three portions;—that which is immediately imbedded in the surrounding integument, to which, from habit, we give the name root; the central portion, called the body; and the extreme end, which is called the top. It is to be observed that in the toe the centre strictly adheres to the subjacent tissue, whilst the root is shut within two laminæ of the skin, although it does not enter into immediate contact with either of them. They appear to belong to the epidermis, and to arise from it, and they are totally devoid of all those vessels and nerves which usually enter into the formation of organized matter; if by any event the epidermis is destroyed, the nails suffer with it, and complete exfoliation occurs. I know not that any of the circumstances connected with their growth and development demands from me much consideration; I would only direct attention to the necessity that exists of watching them, to prevent the annoyances to which they give rise.

It is always necessary for those whose duty calls upon them to watch over the proper development of the toes, to look to the healthy expansion of the nail as the principal object of their attention, after guarding against injudicious pressure, for upon this depends much more of the free exercise of the feet than might at first be imagined. If the nails are healthfully developed, they prevent much mischief to the tender extremities of the toes, to which they form a protecting shield. In our various positions of life, the foot is necessarily the avant-coureur to the rest of the frame, and is therefore more exposed to accidents, to hurts, to bruises, than any other portion of the body, and it often forms a certain defence. It has been justly said, "that a man without good toe nails is fit for nothing in life, not even for an omnibus." He who once has had tender toes, and has found how much he has to endure from such an exposure in a public conveyance, will best find an answer to such a question. A very slight injury to the toe, divested of its natural protection, will cause extreme pain, and even lock-jaw and death have rapidly followed upon the wound of nerves which have been thus exposed. The too rapid growth of the nail may become a source of much inconvenience, more especially if the tendency be laterally, when the neighbouring toe becomes the sufferer; it is of course a less inconvenience, if instead of this the nail goes on increasing its apex, but if it grows thus it is not without its inconvenience; sometimes it doubles itself up, or grows backwards, or pushes itself into the lateral flesh; at others it splits, breaks, thickens, exfoliates; indeed, when once a deviation has begun, it is difficult to say what turn it may take, and to what irregularity it may lead. The growing into the flesh on the side is one of the evils to which the great toe nail is especially liable, although it sometimes from neglect occurs even in the nails of the hands; for all these varied inconveniences the practitioner must be prepared, and he must bear in mind that almost every case requires a different mode of treatment, and that it is quite out of the question to attempt to lay down general laws; in some instances the consequence is but slight, whilst in others dangers of no trifling importance may present themselves. Inflammation will arise sometimes of a serious aspect, for it is to be remembered that in affections of the feet, however apparently trifling, serious symptoms may set in, which under ordinary circumstances would not occur. It is not long since a nobleman—the late Earl of Darnley—distinguished for his high state of health, who had shown that his constitution could withstand the ordinary shocks to which man is liable, was a corpse in a few hours from such a wound near the toe nail, as would have passed unnoticed in the neighbourhood of the vital parts of the frame.

The more striking affections of the nails seem to depend upon a more rapid growth than nature is capable of sustaining, or of such alterations in their structure as leads to a change in their constituent parts, or to their becoming productive of mechanical injury to surrounding tissues. In the first instance we find them rapidly progressing, then splitting, cracking, or exfoliating; in the second, we observe them imperfectly formed, or subject to various diseases; and, in the third, they grow backwards, become imbedded in the side, or lead to various deformities, which demand mechanical skill to cure them. In both the first instances we have to examine whether there may not be some constitutional states which are productive of various alterations in the economy, rendering the cases much more difficult of treatment than they otherwise would be. Of mechanical injuries, which often cause the total loss of nail, there is much to be considered; but the nature of the accident must entirely regulate the treatment, so that it would be utterly impossible to lay down general rules. The loss of the nail from a bruise, from a burn, from exposure to cold, demands such exceedingly different treatment, that no general laws could be laid down; and to enter into them particularly would demand a much greater degree of minuteness than my limits would possibly allow. In cold climates, even in the north of Germany, so much will the temperature affect the minute circulation through the vessels of the extremities, that after many hours' exposure to intense cold the nails will be loosened from the epidermis, and come away unchanged. The great object which should always be had in view, under such circumstances, is the reproduction of the nail; and it is a singular fact, that an annual growth and falling off will often occur for several years, until at last a permanent development takes place, when they remain unchanged, and without any apparent alteration in their shape and form. The tendency to the reproduction of the nails is a striking feature in their economy, and though sometimes, where a loss of blood has originally attended upon it, and such a seemingly morbific action has been set up in the integuments, still the effort of nature, assisted by art, has overcome all difficulties, and led to their complete re-establishment.

The periodical attention to the state of the growth of the nails is what I would more immediately insist upon, and I recommend every one to find some person in whom he can place confidence to inspect his feet two or three times in the course of the year. However attentive a man is to the cleanliness of his person, however watchful over the occasional paring his nails, yet alterations go on stealthily, and creep upon him before he is aware that there is the slightest deviation from the ordinary course. The extreme points of the feet scarcely come within the scope of vision, and few men can form a correct judgment for themselves of what may be taking place; they are satisfied if they feel no inconvenience, and flatter themselves that as things have always gone on well that they will do so always; but there are a variety of changes eternally taking place in a man's person, of which he is the last to be cognizant. He knows not that he is growing older, that the system of to-day is somewhat different from that of yesterday, and that it is necessary to be on his guard for to-morrow. I am recommending prevention; I am not now speaking of cure; but this I must say, that one-half of the maladies which it has been my lot to have witnessed might have been prevented had ordinary care been taken. If alterations occur in the various states and stages of human life, in features, in the strength of the muscular system, in the vigour of the senses,—is it not likely that the same change takes place in all the more minute circumstances of life; and that in the nails singular variations occur, the slightest observation certainly proves. They are soft in infancy, and tinged with red, whilst in youth they have spots of white; in later life they assume a purple hue; but look at them after a fever, or after any severe trial of the constitution, they have become soft and pale, are thin at the top and at the edges, and sometimes fall off. Look at them in the incipient consumption, their rapid growth, their similarity to the beak of a bird. Again, observe how they betray the blood that circulates in the veins! Not all the salt to be found in the ocean would wash away the little black spot that tells us the negro blood has at some time or other been infused into the European. The nails betray the secret, and the initiated is often made acquainted through them with secrets that he could by no other means have fathomed.

The great desideratum is to render the top of the nail round, to prevent the sides growing into the circumjacent flesh, and to keep the root firmly and properly embedded in the folds of the epidermis; the spongy substance which shoots out should be pressed down, taking care not to remove it, for nature seems to have intended it as a protection to the quick. The superfluous skin requires to be taken away, and a regular semicircle should be formed. The nails will sometimes split in a manner that will require the assistance of an experienced operator, for external substances may add to the mischief, and the simpler means will be of no avail; and it may become necessary to wear for some days a guard, to prevent further mischief. If the nails grow into the flesh, it will also be generally necessary to have assistance, for the irritation may be sufficient to excite inflammation, which may run on to suppuration, or the formation of fungous excrescences, which are not so easy of cure as may at first be conceived. The nail must sometimes be cut down to the root. Tearing the nails is a very bad practice, and can never be required as long as a knife or a pair of scissors can be obtained; pain, heat, and much irritation often follow upon this thoughtless proceeding, which would be necessarily avoided if that regularity of attention which I would strongly inculcate were persevered in. The loosened nail—the false nail, as it is termed—demands more care than it generally receives. It would be useless for me to enter upon the treatment, for the cases vary very much, two being scarcely alike, and demand varied treatment; generally, however, cutting carefully and tenderly away all diseased portions, and separating the growing nail from the subjacent skin, is required. The whitlow is a disease which sometimes assumes a very serious character, and is dependent upon inattention to the state of the nails, under which a swelling takes place; an abscess is formed, the serum of which is of a singular character, becoming highly acrid, sometimes even corroding the periosteum, and acting upon the bones so as to produce caries. Sometimes great constitutional disturbance accompanies them; the glands sympathize and become painfully tumid. The treatment then must be decisive; the serous fluid must be evacuated by the lancet before it has had time to burrow deeply; leeches have been recommended, but they seldom are serviceable; cold lotions, and applications of the preparation of lead, are required to the fingers. It may be generally concluded that, when they make their appearance, there is a want of tone which can only be imparted by medical advice and attention to diet.

CHAPTER VIII.

CHILBLAINS are the maladies of youth, and sometimes more difficult to be borne than evils which affect us at a later period. Endurance and philosophy are the results of experience, and we quietly submit to affections which are beyond the reach of art. This pest of youth is a source of much greater pain than we are aware of, for even those who have most acutely suffered, forget, as objects crowd upon their memory, the severe trials of their early life, the tears they have shed, the itching they have endured, the throbbing, the burning, the miseries of the sleepless night produced in the school day by those inveterate foes to ease and tranquillity—chilblains. These tumors, marked by all the characters which have been shown to belong to inflammation, are most painfully felt in early life, when, from the activity of the circulation, the minutest artery of the integument becomes injected with blood; each nerve, however minute, is pressed upon, and the distension of the tissue is such that it is almost insupportable. Then comes the venous retardation, with all its concomitant evils, and ulcerations of the most fearful kind arise. Although some of the most sensitive parts of the body—such as the lips, ears, nose, and hands, may become the seat of chilblains, I have solely to consider them as affecting the feet, and it is upon the toes or upon the heels that they are more generally found, assuming a variety of appearances, which, from their familiarity to the greater mass of people, I need not enumerate. Sufficient for me is it to remark, that on their first appearance they are evidently tumors, to which there is a large determination of arterial blood, evidenced by the throbbing, the heat, and by the reddish inflammatory tint; they then become surcharged with venous blood, daily do they become of a darker and purpler hue, troublesome and insupportable itching succeeding to pain; after which another stage is perceptible, when the accumulated blood attempts to throw off a portion of its serous substance, when new and more violent throbbings and pulsations arise, then the epidermis is separated from the tissues beneath, and large or small vesicles are formed, into which an acrid liquor is poured, by whose agency the superincumbent skin is burst, and irregular ulcerations are produced, which, being most extensive, involve every part of the foot, and even at last the bones themselves become the prey to disease. Throughout the whole history of the disease, the physiologist is enabled to trace the efforts made by nature to relieve herself from the aggravated character of the inflammation, and the physiologist could not select a better subject to prove the inherent anxiety of each part of the system to relieve itself from the dangers with which it is threatened. The stages of the affection are strongly marked, and the remedies for each are well indicated. At the same time it is a matter of regret that they have been neglected even by the most observant surgeons; and means have been had recourse to in one stage unsuccessfully, which, had they been taken when absolutely required, would have been at once useful and proper. The chilblain, if duly watched, is very easy of cure, and much suffering to the most helpless part of the community would be spared if a little attention were paid. Indeed, a school in which chilblains are allowed to run to a certain stage must be badly regulated, and there must be neglect in a department of the utmost importance in the economy of education. For it is not the mind alone which is to be rendered excellent, the body must meet with its due attention, and deformity of the one will soon tend to the debility and destruction of the other.

It is to be regretted that in schools there is so much carelessness as to the state of young people committed to the charge of persons who, however anxious they may be as to the progress of the mind, forget that the body has its claims to watchfulness and attention. At the coming on of the winter every parent and instructor should take care that the clothing be properly adapted to the wants of the young,—warm stockings and thick gloves more especially should be provided. Sudden transitions from heat to cold should be guarded against; ablution with warm water should be followed by gentle friction; wet shoes ought always to be quickly changed; gentle exercise should be insisted upon; dancing ought to be encouraged, and more especially at home, where neither change of dress nor sudden exposure to heat or cold are likely to be encountered, whilst the dance upon the carpet is preferable to the bare boards which the ball room offers. The occasionally rubbing the feet with eau de Cologne, aromatic vinegar, or brandy properly diluted, will be found very serviceable. With such attention chilblains may be altogether kept off, even where there is a strong predisposition to them; but these precautions are not to be followed only for a short time and then forgotten, they are to be persevered in with punctuality and determination. Twice in each week an examination should be made, and if there be a tendency to inflammation, lotions consisting of camphor mixture, lotions of acetate of ammonia, of diacetate of lead, and of those sedative applications which are ordinarily employed for the resolution of inflammation, avoiding all narcotic sedatives, for their external application is more prejudicial than advantageous. Sea water, or a solution of salt, will sometimes be productive of great good; astringent washes of zinc, and of alum, may also be used. In the second stage, and during the retardation of the venous blood, stimulants are required; and we find turpentine, liquor ammonia, cantharides, adapted for them. Previous to this leeches may be used, but I am not an advocate for their employment without due consideration, for in many instances they do not act as in general cases of local inflammation; for there is again a very rapid influx of blood into the capillary vessels, besides which there is often an intolerable itching left behind, which keeps up a fearful state of irritation. The production of cold, by the evaporation of ether, by the use of spirit, or the immediate application of ice, not only gives temporary relief, but permanent, if it be persevered in for some time; compresses, dipped in cold lotions, should be unremittingly kept upon the part affected until the redness, heat, and swelling have disappeared. The warm fomentations, such as decoctions of poppies, of chamomile flowers, of turnips, are occasionally successful, but I by no means recommend them, for I have been uniformly successful in the removal of chilblains in their inflammatory stage by means of cold lotions.

When ulceration has taken place we shall find that much more difficulty arises than could have been suspected, and very quickly will the constitution sympathize, if we are not able to check its progress. We must first enjoin absolute rest; the horizontal position must be maintained, and any exposure to heat or to cold avoided, all the applications which science has discovered will be useless without these primary regulations. Emollient cataplasms, sedative liniments, are in the first instance necessary for the alleviation of pain. We then must have recourse to such measures as the particular case may require; sometimes gentle stimulants, at other times more active ones, are necessary; we have in the first instance cantharides, ammonia, nitrate of silver, to depend upon; in the second, camphorated lotions, the balsams, mustard; but it is not requisite I should enter into details, for they must so much depend upon the precise nature of the affection. The regimen must be most cautiously watched, for the local applications will be hardly serviceable unless the diet be abstemious, and the system properly regulated. It is only now and then that I am called upon to witness those deplorable cases, which were so common in former days, where mortification rapidly advanced, where bark, where antiseptics, were absolutely necessary; for, fortunately for the human race, these evils have nearly disappeared, at least amongst the classes of society which I am most commonly called on to attend. The humblest classes are by the watchfulness of nature generally free from the disorder in the worst stages, for their feet become hardened by the exercise they take, by their exposure to the vicissitudes of weather, and their superficial coverings are generally so thickened and hardened as to free them from the evils to which the more delicate are exposed. We now seldom see constitutions so tainted as to yield to chilblains, and to be so exhausted as to be almost incapable of assisting art in healing them; for, with proper attention, we are now enabled to meet every case that presents itself, and although some little time may be demanded, we are generally successful. Oftentimes, indeed, there is a greater prolongation of time for cure than satisfies the anxieties of friends. This, however, is the case where there is some constitutional taint — where there is a scrofulous diathesis. This state of ill-health was, I understand, formerly much more prevalent in England than it now is. Medical treatment in early life, good food, and proper clothing, have had a material influence upon it; and I am too happy to say that cases such as are described by the older surgical authors, now rarely make their appearance.

The gangrene, or mortification of the chilblain, is the separation of the part which dies from the living portion by a process which nature sets up for the purpose of protecting herself from infection. The stages are beautifully defined from the moment when sensibility gradually is lost to that when fresh substance is formed,— the changes of the tint of the flesh from brown to a black or livid green, the line of demarcation between the morbid portion and the organized circle of life by which it is surrounded, are strikingly visible, and the remedial agents which are to be employed must be strictly adapted to the efforts of nature. The system throughout is to be supported; proper local applications must stimulate the torpid powers, and every circumstance must be duly and thoroughly attended to. The application of charcoal, of the chlorurets of lime and of soda, the use of bark, of steel, of wine, of opium, must be the general remedial agents; nor must we expect that we can at once check the progress of the complaint, for when once the mortification has commenced, it will run its general course, the only duty of the medical man being to watch the indications of nature, and to be enabled to render her that assistance which she may require, always bearing in mind neither to be too meddlesome nor too indolent in our treatment,—the happy art being to steer between the two extremes.

CHAPTER IX.

THE hand becomes next the object of my examination. It will be remembered that the Earl of Bridgewater left by his will, in the year 1825, eight thousand pounds to be given to such person or persons who would write works illustrative of the power, wisdom, and goodness of God, as manifested in the Creation; and amongst the points selected was the construction of the hand of man. The President of the Royal Society appointed the late Sir Charles Bell to write the treatise, which he did, under the title of "The Hand, its Mechanism and vital Endowments," as evincing design, and for which he received one thousand pounds. He published it in 1837. To those who are familiar with the anatomical writings of that distinguished professor, there is less of novelty than to the public at large, for we perceive throughout it the same train of reflection which he has given us in his three volumes of anatomy, and in his papers upon the nervous system, read before the Royal Societies of London and of Edinburgh. It would be a matter of presumption on my part to attempt to discuss the opinions of one who, familiar with physiology and comparative anatomy, has entered into a philosophic inquiry into the physical properties, the mechanical construction, and the singular endowment of this most inportant organ of the human frame. I must confine my own observations to the means by which it may be enabled to carry out the objects, not for which it was originally designed, but for which, according to the customs and manners of polished society, it is to be employed. It is not for me to examine it, as the organ by which so many important actions are to be performed. It is not as covered with the coarse skin which enables the operator to perform so many manipulations, with a hardened cuticle which prevents too much sensibility, or with nails capable of grasping objects, it is as covered with a delicate epidermis, with soft integuments under it, for the purpose of increasing the power of sensation, and for that delicacy of touch which affords pleasure, and the capability of receiving transient impressions. Attention to the state of the skin of the hands, to the nails, and to the formation of the fingers, is rarely given at that time of life when the system is developing itself; and yet there is much more necessity for it than we are willing to allow; upon their management much of the power of the artist depends. The painter, the sculptor, who has pliable and flexible hands, who has delicacy of touch, and quickness of sensation, will be superior to him who has the greater power of conception and of invention. The organization of the hand may be perfect as to its muscular power, may be endowed with a high degree of elasticity; but if, besides this, there is not all that can be given to it, by unremitting watchfulness of defects, by constant cleanliness, and careful preservation of the skin and nails, not only will there be clumsiness in action, but there will be imperfection in the sensation and in the power of construction. There are occupations in life which are entirely dependent upon the sensibility of the nerves of touch, yet how little are those who follow them aware that, by attention and management, they are either to be heightened or diminished.

The same dermoid coverings which exist in the foot and the rest of the human body are found extended over the whole of the hand, modified according to the circumstances in which each individual is placed. The epidermis has the same functions to perform; it is the guard and protector of the subjacent tissue, and is thick or thin, according to the uses which are made of the hand. In some persons it is exquisitely soft and thin, conveying the sensation of touch with rapidity and intensity; in others, it is remarkably thick and hard, and capable of resisting external impression. This apparatus, too, differs according to the sensibility of the different parts of the hand. At the tops of the fingers, there are minute spiral ridges, having depressed lines, which are also marked in the under surface, and in these are lodged the extreme ends of nerves, formed into a pulpy mass. At the verge of the finger is situated the nail, a continuation of the cuticle, of excessive thickness, formed into a fold; its origin has been a subject of much discussion, some persons entertaining the belief that it is a condensation of the rete mucosum ; and it is by it, as I have before observed, that we are enabled, by means of the tinge of black which remains from generation to generation, to ascertain whether any negro blood flows through the veins of an individual. In the West Indies and in the United States, where there is great discrimination of what is called a taint in the blood, the proof is supposed to be decisive if the root of the nail exhibit the slightest approximation to a dark hue. The epidermis permits the perspiration to exude through it, and has a very striking influence in rendering the body cool or warm; the perspiration is of considerable importance to the state of health, and the skilful physician draws his indications of the health or disease of an individual from its state. A warm hand, even if covered with a gentle dew, is necessary in some climates, whilst the cold clammy moisture is to be avoided. In winter, the caloric is rapidly absorbed by the atmosphere, and cold generated throughout the whole of the body. If the hand be not properly protected, and if the vascular surface under the epidermis be deprived of its proper heat, sensation is lost; that state of numbness is produced which not only has an influence upon the muscular fibre but upon the secretions of the body, some of which are rapidly diminished, whilst others, on the other hand, are inordinately increased.

If on the one hand roughness of the cuticle on the palm of the hand and the fingers is to be avoided, so likewise is too much delicacy. We are sometimes rendered insensible to the smoothness of some surfaces, for by the great smoothness of the skin we are unable to grasp objects with firmness. Fortunately, however, the habits of society do not demand the steady and decisive grasp which the mechanic and the labourer find essentially necessary in their occupations. There is, generally speaking, too little attention paid to the state of the hands and fingers; all that is thought of is cleanliness, and an occasional paring of the nails; but it would be as well if, from an early period, care was taken of the manner of the development of the hands, so that they may acquire beauty of shape, flexibility, and muscular power. The shape of the fingers will be found materially to influence the sense of touch; they should be rendered tapering, whilst the extreme end must, in the lower part, be allowed a full development, so that a sort of soft cushion may exist, formed of the sentient nerves, covered over with a fine elastic epidermis. This organization is necessary for the acuteness of touch, whilst the nails should be firm and hard shields for the upper surface: the healthy state of the membrane is to be preserved by constant ablution, by the occasional use of sand soap, by gentle friction with the flesh brush, by gloves properly adapted to the warmth or cold of the weather, and by the occasional passing the hand frequently through the air, as in fanning. Nothing can be more injurious than the system which has been recommended for the purpose of producing a temporary whiteness and delicacy of the hand and arm, and which consists in holding the arm in an upright position for a considerable length of time, and even, as it has been asserted, of tying them in that position for hours. It is true that the cuticular circulation is for a time checked in the very minute branches of the vascular system, but it soon returns, and there is often a venous blueness produced by the reaction, infinitely more disagreeable to the eye than the redness which was complained of. Many cosmetics have been tried, but with little or no good effect, and they sometimes have been productive of mischief, more especially those which have been composed of preparations of lead, for whatever may be asserted by chemists as to the harmlessness of some of the compounds of that metal, there are many instances on record of irretrievable paralysis produced by them, and more especially where the epidermis has been removed.

The nails are to be watched from an early period of youth, by those parents who are anxious to do their duty to their families, and it is a subject of much regret that at schools they are so constantly neglected. I would not have a boy effeminate or a coxcomb, but he should be instructed in those little duties that render his future life more agreeable to him, and that at last grow into habits, which become of importance to him when old age, with all its want of comforts, creeps on. The nails are never to be bitten or torn off, they are to be kept free from all sort of dirt and sordes, whose accumulation blocks up the termination of the nerves, impedes a free circulation of the blood, and thus impairs the sense of touch, if not the general health. The free transpiration through the skin is often impeded by inattention to the nails. What the connexion between the nails and the diseases of the human system depends upon, it is not for me to explain, that I must leave to the pathologist; but every attentive observer of nature is aware that there is some latent communication. The consumptive patient exhibits the peculiar state of nail by which the physician knows that the lungs are affected; nay, nosologists have taken it as one of their characteristic marks of the worst stage of phthisis. A child who has a scrofulous habit will have such brittle nails that they will break before they attain any strength. The red deeply tinged nail is found concomitant with gout; the blue, with asthma; in some fevers they become pale and thin. In the cold stage of an intermittent fever they almost seem shrivelled up, whilst in the hot they are larger than ordinary. It therefore becomes the bounden duty of all to be attentive even to those minutiæ which escape observation generally. It is useless for me to attempt to determine the exact length to which the nail should be suffered to grow, but I would recommend that a certain day be fixed in each week for attention to them; such regularity is always attended with great advantages, the system acquires as it were a periodicity, besides which it is remembered, and comes into the usual economy of life. Where this is the case, too, there will never be those ragged integuments, which are oftener the source of mischief than is believed, for by simply covering a denuded spot by common court-plaster, absorption will be prevented. The nail brush should frequently be used, and the removal of any extraneous matter be managed by blunt instruments, for knives and pointed scissors are likely to wound and irritate the sentient extremities; and besides this, the nail is not unfrequently so loosened, that it does not retain its proper hold in the rest of the integuments.

Accustomed to so many of the phenomena of life as we are, some of the most extraordinary pass by us completely unnoticed, because our minds are more engrossed with those which seem to be the most difficult to understand. The performance of a young child upon the pianoforte is an object of such daily occurrence that we are not struck with any emotions of surprise or admiration; yet a moment's reflection would show us what numerous duties the nerves, the muscles, and the mind are called upon at the same moment to perform. The eye must seize with rapidity all the variations of notes, time, and rhythm, whilst the fingers must strike the keys with instantaneous motion. There must be a perfect correspondence between the intellect and the muscular power; the ear must also be alive to every modification of sound; yet there must appear no labour, no hurry, no difficulty. Sensibility the most delicate is alive to every want of consonance of mind and body. The training the hand to this obedience demands, in many instances, much time, whilst some seem to have an intuitive power of expressing harmony,—they have a natural gift by which, in the most orderly and systematic manner, they command the instrument on which they play. It is not for me to enter upon the field which more immediately belongs to the professor of music, but I would observe that in the greater number of instances there is too little attention paid to the shape and form of the fingers and thumb of individuals —their power of expansion, of action, their flexibility, and their elasticity. Some young persons are called upon to use muscular power of which they are incapable. They have placed before them pieces of music, admirably adapted, doubtless, for the gigantic grasp of some artist who has devoted his life to his art; but instructors are forgetful of the utter impossibility of stretching the muscles, ignorant of the tendons which are called into play, or the fascia that prevents the effort from being carried into execution. I would strongly recommend every parent and guardian, and certainly every superintendent of a school, to become familiar with the general anatomy of the hand, to learn what form and configuration prevent a child from making such progress as the eager ambition of fond parents may desire. Not only do they look for impossibilities, but they may be the cause of the production of future mischief. The hand may lose much of its natural power; nay, be so harassed by vain efforts as to become incapable of performing many of the offices required. Writing may become so painful as to be almost abandoned; besides which, upon the slightest exertion fatigue will supervene. The weakness of wrist so often complained of amongst ladies may not unfrequently be traced to the undue muscular exercise in early life.

Whilst each of the fingers plays its part in the general economy, serving to give flexibility, tenacity, firmness, and strength to the hand, the thumb is in itself an instance of wondrous workmanship, which exhibits that everything has been designed for the use of man, with a providential care for his well-being. Being placed in immediate opposition to the fingers, it is enabled to assist them in holding and grasping objects. It renders the hand more powerful, more useful, than the claws, the hoofs, the horns, the talons, the spurs, and the beaks of other created beings; and as our venerable naturalist Ray has observed, "Man hath none of all these, but is weak and feeble, and sent unarmed into the world:—why, a hand, with reason to use it, supplies the use of all these." The various directions in which the thumb acts gives to it power in the different purposes of life; it is of exceeding strength, and rolls widely and freely. Its tendons and joints, together with its peculiar bursa, are all most ingeniously contrived, and enable us as well to exert power in heaving an anchor or delicacy in picking up a needle. It is, of all the organs we possess, the one we most frequently call into action, and the one which seems less liable to fatigue. Not only are all the labours of man dependent on it—for neither could he dig, nor spin, nor plant, nor weave without it—but those intellectual occupations which form the source of his superiority must altogether cease. The pen is guided by the incessant motion of this little agent, which has conveyed from age to age the learning of the wise and the good, and diffused a knowledge of all that has been observed. Of the hand we do not avail ourselves, as do some of the nations of the globe, for assistance in speech. Quintilian has, in a few powerful words, expressed the uses to which the Romans applied the hand. He says:—"Other parts assist the speaker, but these, if I may use the expression, speak themselves; by these we demand, we promise, we call, we dismiss, we threaten, we supplicate, we hate, we fear; joy, sorrow, doubt, confession, repentance, sufficiency, plenty, number, time, we show." At this day both the Roman and the Neapolitan are remarkable for their gestures; whole conversations pass, games are played, and the varying passions delineated by the thumb and the fingers. Their expressive countenances oftentimes speak less than do these organs. They seem to be enabled to convey every idea that flashes across the mind; and whether he who accomplishes his end, or he who comprehends the ever-varying motion, be the most ingenious, it is most difficult to understand.

The thumb is so essentially necessary to the power of man, that were it wanting he would be incapable of following any of those pursuits in which he is engaged; without that fleshy protuberance which rises on the last joint, he would be almost helpless. The anatomist, once the great leader of the schools of surgery, Albinus, has characterized the thumb as a small hand, the assistant of the greater "manus parva majori adjutrix." We may generally judge of the dexterity of a man by the shape of his thumb, and the pretended fortune-tellers are fully alive to this fact when they pronounce, on examining the hand, the degree of superiority which a man has attained as a workman. The coarseness or delicacy of the skin, the shape of the fingers, and the form of the thumb, indicate many circumstances which the inexperienced observer passes over. The different length of the fingers is another provision of nature; it is absolutely necessary for many of the manipulations that this should be the case; were it not so, the art of writing, which has delighted us with the works of Byron, of Walter Scott, or of a Schiller, a Goethe, a Homer, or Milton, could not have been followed; for take the means of writing, the pen grasped by the thumb and the indicator finger, rests upon the very termination of the middle finger, which again receives support from the other two fingers,—so is it with every one of the fine arts, the brush could not be held by the painter, nor the chisel by the sculptor, were the fingers of an equal length. But the numerous illustrations of which the subject admits must not now detain me; my object is rather to show that attention to what nature demands of us should be more generally given than it is, and that we should carefully learn the end and aims of our great Artificer, because from them we ascertain what is best to be done for the proper health and due preservation of each part of the human structure, and that we should be enabled not only to counteract many deviations from a normal state, but that we have it in our power to render our original gifts more available, and thus by early education and watchfulness we shall be enabled to turn them to greater account, not only for our own benefit, but for that of society at large.

Various have been the cosmetics, washes, tinctures, soaps, unguents, "et hoc genus omne," with which the learned as well as the unlearned have tried to give a delicate whiteness to the hands and arms; few of these things possess much value except as simple detergents, and as keeping the surface from impurities, or gently increasing the perspiration. Some of the common vegetables,—such as horse-radish, house-leek, turnips, apples—have been recommended, either in the form of cataplasm, or the juice extracted from them; and various are the recipes which are found in the old herbalists, each of which has some respectable authority for its employment. It would be useless for me to discuss the subject, because although I have found many very useful where there has been want of attention, and various unseemly affections have made their appearance under the form of pimples, blotches, redness, scurf, yet each case requires its own peculiar treatment, and oftentimes the constitution is much in fault. A very excellent wash is formed of the tincture of Benjamin, in rose or in distilled water; the balsam of Peru, with yolk of egg, or mucilage of gum arabic, in some instances sulphate of zinc, oxide of bismuth, and others of the metallic salts, may be judiciously employed; but as none of these are to be used without knowing the exact state of the skin, I shall not enter into details which cannot be fully borne out by the experience which is necessary. A temporary whiteness of the hands ought not to be sought after, because it is always followed by lasting deterioration of the skin. If by care and attention we can obtain that which constitutes beauty, it is both right and honourable to do everything that lays within our power, but a mere transient effect should not be produced, more especially when in the greater number of instances it leads to mischief.

I have pointed out the necessity of attention to the proper coverings for the feet, and a few words upon those of the hand may be admissible, although there is not so much dependent upon them. Gloves should be worn according to the state of the weather: a thin glove in winter will be the cause of redness and of discoloration, whilst a hot one in summer will bring with it increased perspiration and eruptions. Those lined with lamb's wool and warm materials, which are so efficient in December, will be quite out of the question in August. The best material for gloves at all times is silk; less so, however, in the midst of summer. The soft leather gloves are well known to be preferable to all others, and therefore I will only further say, that a change of the materials of gloves occasionally is of great service. Many incipient eruptions and discolorations vanish upon substituting for a few days different gloves from those which have been generally worn, and a change of temperature being superinduced, relieves the system also from many of those temporary inconveniences arising from an alteration in the state of the perspiration; it is not for me to point out the varieties which present themselves; the subject would occupy a vast deal more space than I can give it, and fortunately the best works in surgery may be consulted by those who are desirous to pursue the subject further. My great desire is to impress upon the minds of mothers and guardians the importance of an early attention to the comforts of the young; for by such means will the worst cases be avoided. Having promised (page 17) to give, in an Appendix, a brief view of the anatomy of the human foot, I have added a concluding chapter, taken from the "Practical Exposition of the Human Foot," written by me some time since.

APPENDIX.

FROM THE

PRACTICAL EXPOSITION OF THE HUMAN FOOT.

CHAPTER X.

THE structure of the human foot is exceedingly beautiful, and well worthy the study of all who love to watch the never-ending wonders of our fabric, each of which seems to have been framed to lead us on to further inquiries. Whenever we examine anatomically any apparatus, and study for what the different contrivances are manifestly intended, we are struck with the simplicity even of apparently the most complicated arrangements. We see that were the organ differently made, it could not adapt itself to all the purposes for which it is destined. That thirty-six bones and that thirty-six joints should enter into the composition of the human foot seems at first to be too bounteous a gift, and that the very number of parts of which such a machine is composed would lead to constant derangements, whilst at the same time all that is performed could be effected at a less expenditure of mechanism; but were the foot formed of one solid bone, however capable it might be of supporting the human body, it would be devoid of that flexibility, elasticity, freedom, and power which give ease of motion, capability of exertion, and elegance of gait to man. The whole fabric of these bones and of these joints is singularly instructive. Each joint unites two bones in such a manner that they are not in immediate contact, each articulating surface is covered with elastic cartilage; its surface is perfectly smooth, being lubricated by an oily fluid called the synovia, covered over by a delicate membrane, extending from bone to bone. This covering or capsule has external to it a strong ligament attached from point to point of each bone, binding them firmly together without impeding in any way their motion. Such numerous joints cannot fail to give a degree of flexibility to the bones which could in no other way be obtained; and were the invention of the most ingenious of men to be ransacked for the purpose of discovering any more perfect contrivance, I am persuaded that it could not approach at the longest interval the machine destined for such a variety of motions and of actions. Whilst the junction of the foot to the bones of the leg demands the most minute inquiry to estimate the beauty of the contrivances which have been carried out, I will for the present moment confine myself to the osteological anatomy of the foot, describing the thirty-six bones of which it is formed and their various connexions with each other.

It has been very properly observed that the foot is the true basis on which our whole machine is supported, and that a sculptor would be working in vain were he to rest his statue on a round and movable foundation; it would undoubtedly fall and be broken to pieces. In order to illustrate the wonderful mechanism of the foot, its muscles, tendons, and its bones, it would be but necessary to mark the evolutions on the toe of one of our celebrated dancers, and observe how the pirouette is performed. The preservation of perpendicularity, of a graceful equilibrium, a picturesque attitude, and a classic arabesque, are to be combined with energetic execution and muscular strength, whilst the whole body is revolving round upon the toe. A pirouette, to be elegantly performed, requires the dancer to turn round not only on one leg, but upon two toes, without the slightest jerk of the body, several times. Not only must there be an unshaken equilibrium, but the position of the arms must be so managed as to maintain the line of gravity with gracefulness. The imitation of some of the statues of antiquity shows what dependence on anatomical structure dancers must have. Of these the most striking is the representation of "Mercury new lighted on a heaven-kissing hill." Unless the foot is perfectly formed this is impossible. The body leans forward, supported entirely on the toe of the foot; the leg that is in attitude must be bent; the right arm is elevated in the air; the left, stretched out, holds the caduceus; the whole frame is rapidly revolved; the movement must appear perfectly natural and unconstrained, every apparent effort to counterpoise the body spoils the whole effect. The dancer has to expand all his toes to make them as it were roots, which hold him to the spot; if he does not do so, his foot loses its natural appearance, a wavering motion is produced, which results from the convexity of the toes, vacillation occurs, the equilibrium is lost, and the whole performance is ridiculous. But however flexible the joints of the foot have become by the constant practice of the dancer, and the freedom of motion may almost equal that of the hand, it does not add to the beauty of the gait in common walking; on the contrary, we are astonished sometimes to observe the tottering steps of the dancer whom we have admired on the stage, and whilst we learn of what the human machine is capable, we do not recommend its education to unnatural positions and useless deviations from its ordinary actions. The foot is so to be regulated that a steady, graceful movement and carriage of the body are the results, and for the ordinary exercise, strength, and flexibility; these cannot exist where there is any mechanical impediment arising out of those alterations of structure, which it is the duty of the Chiropodist to watch over and to prevent. It would appear almost absurd to recommend the general reader to observe the beautiful display made in the ballet by the accomplished dancer, but any one who wishes to become familiar with the structure which Nature has so harmoniously and exquisitely framed will find in dancing on the stage the finest illustrations. The steps, the motions, the attitudes, exhibit in the utmost perfection the capabilities of the muscular system. The enjoyment which is to be derived from the display of grace and elegance will be much heightened by the study of the anatomical structure which admits of it. It is the subjection of the foot, the legs, the arms, and the body, to certain and definite rules, that constitutes greatness in the art. Doubtless the ars saltationis of the Romans was but leaps, tumbling, and grotesque exertions of the limbs and the body. Extravagant contortions, uncouth motions, and unmeaning attitudes have long been banished from the schools of art, and in their place we have a systematic arrangement of every part of the body in strict harmony, and in accurate unison with the cadence of time and the accompanying music. The nobler works of the painter and the sculptor are studied,—groups such as those which have emanated from the most inventive genius, are placed before us. To Italy, the birthplace of all that is captivating in art, we are indebted for the ballet as it is at present before us, and we acknowledge that it is invested with a character which renders it not unworthy the most civilized nations. Noverre was the first dancer who attempted to improve the principles and powers of the art, by writing a treatise containing instructions which every aspirant to greatness in that art should read. Nor were the philosophers who wrote the French Encyclopædia unmindful of the influence which dancing has upon a polished nation. Blasis has since that time given to the amateurs and professors of the art a work full of sensible observations on its theory and its practice. He has shown what many and what varied qualities are necessary to form a perfect dancer; and he has forcibly dwelt upon the attention which should be paid, by each person anxious to excel, upon the peculiarities which mark his formation. He has shown that the defects of different persons, whilst they may altogether prohibit their venturing on one class of performance, may be so managed as to become the source of excellence in another. The make of a person must be studied, the natural construction of his legs and his feet must be carefully observed, for some are so faulty that any attempt to remedy or relieve the defects would be useless, whilst others again have every external qualification, but want the discretion and the taste to develop them. In the different animals inferior to man great is the variety displayed in the formation of the foot. Each family has its own marked characteristic organ, admirably suited to the part he has to play in the great theatre of the world; the mechanism is infinitely varied, and its adaptation for the wants of the animal is always most appropriate. The foot of the horse, the camel, the elephant, has each its own peculiarities, enabling the animal to fulfil the duties which man requires of him; and each seems to exhibit in its structure that he was created to be subservient to a higher being, and to supply his wants and his desires. The more comparative anatomy is studied the more evident is it that the upright figure of man is dependent upon his conformation, and that no animal approaches him in that most striking of his characteristics. The formation of his pelvis, the obliquity of the neck of the thigh-bone, the distances of the trochanters from the sockets, the lar ge muscles of the loins and hips, all are associated with the form of the foot. The Simia Troglodytes, or Chimpanzee, an example of which whilst living was in the Zoological Gardens, and whose skeleton may now be studied in the Museum, comes nearer to the human species than any other being; but it is evident that only for a very short space of time could he sustain the erect position. The deviations from the structure of other skeletons visible in the Marsupial family are well worthy investigation; for we find that there are singularities of formation which enable it to rest in the perpendicular, but this is done by the assistance of its tail, on which, together with its paws, it balances itself as on a tripod. With these two exceptions all animals bend, at all times prone to the earth, and this arises from that conformation which should be thoroughly examined to learn the cause of man's superiority.

The foot of the horse forms a most interesting study as a piece of mechanism. What strength, what power, what elasticity, are there combined! The bones, the ligaments, and the hoof, have configurations adapted for their use which have now very properly been investigated by the veterinary surgeon, who "finds each time he demonstrates the anatomy something new to admire." This subject, which is so much neglected by the surgeon, is considered of importance by the veterinary professors, who have been enabled to obtain a charter for a Royal College, whilst the Chiropodist is looked down upon as practising a branch almost illegitimate and scarcely to be recognized amongst the auxiliary branches of medicine.

The bones of the foot have their own peculiar mechanical construction; indeed, it has justly been observed, "that there is hardly a bone which has not a constitution of its own, or a disposition of material adjusted to its place and its use. The heel bone, the shin bone, the vertebræ, and the bones of the head,—all differ in their mechanical construction." The great object which seems to have been considered in the anatomical structure of the foot is to give perfect security during all the great exertions which it is called on to make in the vast variety of motion of which it is capable. It is equally adapted for walking, for running, for leaping; it is formed for kicking, for grasping; and there are many offices it would perform were it not in civilized society rendered of less use than it is amongst a people living in a state of nature. We shall find that so admirably has Nature contrived her handiwork, that the form of each bone of the foot, of which there are so many, is exactly in unison with the motion to be performed, and that were any part or portion actually different from what we find it, there would be some impediment to the actions which are necessary. The articulations of the bones, too, are equally advantageous. The forms of bones are also so contrived as best to suit the origin and insertion of the various muscles, and their strength and thickness vary according to their relative position and bearing upon these muscles. The constituents, too, of which these bones are formed is another proof, if more were wanting, of singular wisdom in the structure of the bones. The three principles—membrane, phosphate, and cartilage—are so united, that no one is so predominant as to overcome the peculiar characteristic of the other material, but they altogether compose a fabric whose properties are admirably adapted for the machinery which is to be set into motion. If we take advantage of comparative anatomy we are still more struck with the bony part of the man's foot; we see how the shape in each animal tends to illustrate the power, the condition, and the station which it holds in creation. The apparatus with which each is supplied is but such a change as best suits his means of obtaining his food, of defending himself against his enemies, or such motion as he may be called on to make, whether flying or creeping, swimming or burrowing. The geologist can also throw much light on these inquiries, for he finds beneath the surface of the earth remains of extinct races, and a single bone may enable him to judge of the size, the habits, and the residence of the creature. The anatomy of the bones of the foot I will now briefly describe, in order that my exposition may contain that which may be found generally useful.

The instep, or tarsus, is composed of seven bones of some size, irregularly shaped and short.

These are so arranged as to form the strongest support of the body a flexible or elastic arch. The astragalus is the most striking of these bones; together with the bones of the leg, the tibia, and the fibula, it forms the ankle joint. It has a semicircular head forming a complete pulley, whose circle is large; its cartilage is well lubricated, and rolls under the articulating surface of the fibula and tibia, and the groove, from its boat-like shape, into which it enters, is called the scaphoid cavity. The attention of the anatomist is directed to the articulating surfaces; its superior surface, or that which is connected with the scaphoid cavity of the tibia; the internal articulating surface, with the malleolus internus, or the protuberance of the inner ankle; the external articulating surface, with the extremity of the fibula; the inferior and anterior surface, with the os calcis or heel bone; the head or anterior articulating surface, which enters into the concave part of the os naviculare, or scaphoid bone, a smooth surface resting on a portion of ligament between the os calcis and the naviculare, a fossa dividing the inferior articulating surface and a groove in which the capsular ligament is placed. On the inside of the bone is a rough protuberance destined for the deltoid ligament. The os calcis or heel bone forms the back part of the arch on which the body rests. There is an irregular process on the projection in the back which serves as the point of insertion for the tendo Achilles, or, as it was formerly called, the Chorda magna; there are two surfaces covered with cartilage, where it is connected with the astragalus; and another by which it is joined with the os cuboides. On the inside there is a concavity, under which the nerves, the vessels, and the tendons pass forward to the foot; on the outer surface there is a groove, which conveys the tendon of the peronœus longus towards its insertion into the metatarsal bone of the great toe and the cuneiform bone. There is a tubercle internally, to which is attached the ligamentum inter os calcis et naviculare. The os naviculare has a concave surface to receive the head of the astragalus, a flat side slightly irregular for the three cuneiform bones, and a tubercle for the ligament running between it and the os calcis. There are three bones, which, from their wedge-like shape, are called cuneiform; one of these, much larger than the other, being the one on which the great toe stands, is called os cuneiforme magnum; the one in the middle is the smallest, and is called os cuneiforme minimum; the other, os cuneiforme medium; the great toe and the two next are in unison with them. The os cuboides, so called from its cubical form, is on the outer side of the third cuneiform bone, and is articulated with the os calcis. There are two surfaces at its anterior point, for two metatarsal bones; and in its lower surface is a groove, for the tendon of the peronœus longus. It is thrust in between the os calcis and the third cuneiform bone, so as to form an arch within an arch; thus the firm and elastic arch is composed, having ligaments to unite it, a lubricating fluid, and every contrivance to render it the most perfect piece of mechanism with which we are acquainted.

The metatarsus is placed between the tarsus and the bones which form the toes, and is composed of five bones. The general structure of these bones is that on their lower sides, where are the tendons of the toes, they are flattened; that they have a ridge upon their upper surface. Where they approximate to the tarsus, they have broad square surfaces, whilst where they are in contact with the first bones of the toes, they have small heads, the extremities terminate in round balls for insertion into the cavities of the first bones of the toes, and there is a groove for the attachment of the capsule. From the anterior extremities are processes for the attachment of the lateral ligaments of the joints, the particular distinctions of the metatarsal bones are not very striking; it is, however, to be noticed, that the metatarsal bone of the great toe is the shortest, that it has the appearance of greater strength, and that it is largest at its extreme head, whilst the metatarsal bone of the second toe is the longest, the metatarsal bone of the little toe has its head fitted to receive the tendons of the peronœus secundus and tertius muscles. The composition of the tarsus and the metatarsus is such that a double arch is formed, upon which the great mobility of the foot depends, and we have a steady basis upon which the frame rests; from the lowest point of the heel to the ball of the great toe, there is the arch of the sole; the astragalus, resembling the keystone of the arch; and this plays freely between the two bones, the os calcis and the os naviculare; then there is an arch from side to side, formed by the os cuboides and the os cuniforme, and then the tarsal bones form themselves into a third arch; thus have we three arches, of which the bones that form them are closely wedged together, but which, nevertheless, admit of flexibility and elasticity, one arch extending the length of the foot, another its breadth, whilst the third is horizontal. The arch which the mason looks upon as the most perfect form of solidity in building, and of which the stones properly wedged together are the constituent parts, thus exists in the foot; but beyond this, each constituent part of that arch is capable of motion, and as has been observed by one of our highest anatomical authorities, "the foundations of the Eddystone lighthouse are not laid on a better principle; but our admiration is more excited on observing that the bones of the foot are not only wedged together like the courses of stone for resistance, but that solidity is combined with elasticity and lightness;" the strong ligaments which unite the bones give an extraordinary degree of flexibility, allowing a free play to every bone; at the same time there is no visible motion in any one of the joints, but it is generally diffused throughout the whole, each part enabling the foot to act as volition directs, and to perform slow or rapid, cautious or firm, light or decided, movements.

There are six muscles attached to the foot, whose office is that of extensors, and two of flexor muscles; four of the former lie on the back part of the leg, two on the outside, whilst the two flexors are situated on the forepart of the leg. The gastrocnemius, the plantaris, the soleus, and the tibialis posticus are the four first; the peronæus longus and brevis the two next; whilst the tibialis posticus, and the pèronæus tertius are the flexors. The gastrocnemius is that muscle which forms the calf of the leg, from the condyles of the femur it takes its origin, having two large bellies, the innermost of which is the largest, its tendon arising from the back of the inner condyle, and it has also an adhesion to the capsular ligament of the knee; its outer head is not so long, springing from the outer condyle, the two different bellies run close to each other, and meet in the middle of the leg, where they unite firmly, forming a large flat tendon, which, joining with the tendon of the soleus, forms the large tendon called the tendo Achilles, which is inserted into the great process of the os calcis. The soleus has also two heads, one having its origin from the head of the fibula, the other from the tibia they unite, and a large fleshy belly is formed. We shall find that Douglas, the celebrated anatomist, considers these two muscles as forming a quadriceps, or two muscles united with two heads, to which he gives the name of extensor suralis. These muscles are called into action in all the movements of the leg. The plantaris has a fleshy origin from the external condyle of the femur, and is also attached to the capsular ligament of the joint; its tendon takes its course between the inner head of the gastrocnemius and the soleus, and attaches itself to the inner edge and fore part of the tendo Achilles, with which it is inserted into the os calcis. The peronæus longus arises partly tendinous, partly fleshy, from the head of the fibula, and along its ridge to nearly the ankle, having also a small slip from the head of the tibia. Its tendon commences above the middle of the leg, runs down behind the outer ankle, giving to it its form, it passes through a groove in the os calcis, and is inserted in the great cuneiforme bone, and in the metatarsal bone of the great toe. This is a most important muscle in the motion of the foot, and it is by its action that the most striking movements in dancing are performed; it enables the artiste to stand upon her toes, and upon its healthy and regular action depends the power of taking great exercise; the agility of the body is also mainly owing to it. In some parts it is exceedingly thick, immediately under the head of the os cuboides, this is so remarkable as to wear the resemblance of ossification. In its length it is bound down by a strong ligamentous expansion.

The peronœus brevis has its origin from the ridge of the fibula, commencing about one-third down; the tendons of the peronœus longus and brevis accompany each other by the outer ankle, and there the peronœus brevis runs into its separate groove, to be inserted into the metatarsal bone of the little toe and the os cuboides. The peronœus tertius has its origin from the lower half of the fibula; its tendon goes under the annular ligament, on the fore part of the os calcis, to be inserted into the metatarsal bone of the little toe. The tibialis posticus arises from the back of the tibia from its ridge, from the fibula, and from the interosseous ligament; its tendon passes into the groove of the inner ankle, and is inserted into all the bones of the tarsus, sending branches amongst the bones of the tarsus and metatarsus. The tibialis anticus has its origin from the fore part and outside of the tibia, from the head of the fibula, and from the interosseous ligament. Its tendon runs along the side of the foot, and is inserted into the os cuneiforme internum and the metatarsal bone of the great toe.

The flexor longus pollicis arises from three-fourths of the fibula, its tendon passing down behind the inner ankle under the heel bone, between the two sesamoid bones at the root of the great toe, is inserted into its last phalanx; it keeps the toe firm to the ground and also bends it.

The flexor longus digitorum pedis arises from the back of the tibia and from the septum tendinosum; its tendon is formed within two inches of the ankle, and is inserted into the third phalanx of the four toes which they bend.

The flexor accessorius has its origin from the lower part of the heel bone, and is inserted into the tendon of the flexor longus digitorum before it divides into tendons for each toe.

The flexor brevis digitorum arises from the lower part of the heel bone and from the plantar aponeurosis, and is inserted into the second phalanges of the four toes.

The lumbricales have their origin from the tendon of the flexor longus, and are inserted into the sides of the first phalanges.

The extensor longus digitorum pedis arises from the head of the tibia at its outer and fore parts from the whole length of the fibula from the interosseous ligament, the fascia, and is inserted into the first phalanx of the four toes.

The extensor digitorum brevis springs from the outer side and fore part of the heel bone, and from part of the annular ligament, and is inserted into all the phalanges of the toes, with the exception of the little one.

The extensor pollicis proprius arises from the fibula, a little below its head, from the interosseous ligament, and is inserted in the second joint over the toe.

The abductor pollicis arises from the os calcis and from the ligament of the naviculare, and is inserted into the first phalanx of the toe and os sesamoideum.

The flexor brevis pollicis has its origin from the os cuneiforme externum and from the os calcis, and is inserted into the sesamoid bones.

The abductor pollicis arises from the os

calcis, from the cuboides and cuneiforme externum, and is inserted either into the external sesamoid bones or the first bone of the great toe.

The transversalis pedis arises from the fore part of the metatarsal bone of the great toe and the internal sesamoid, and is inserted into the metatarsal bone of the little toe and the ligament of the tarsus.

Abductor minimi digiti, from the os calcis, inserted into the root of the first bone of the little toe.

Flexor brevis minimi digiti arises from the metatarsal bone of the little toe, and is inserted into the first bone of the little toe.

The interossei interni and externi form a web, having their origin in the metatarsal bones, and are inserted in the tendinous aponeurosis.

The toes form the last of the divisions of

the foot, and we find them disposed into three separate bones; they are placed in rows, and to these the term phalanges has been appropriated. But whilst the toes generally have each three phalanges, the great toe has but two. These bones are so made that they have upon their lower side a flattened groove into which the tendons of the last joint of the toes enter. The bones situated nearest the metatarsal bones have their articulating surfaces as deep sockets for their reception, whilst the articulation of the second and third joints are hinge joints. The heads of these bones are large, and they have a lateral projection for the reception of the lateral ligaments. Small bones about the size of the sesamum are found about the toes, one on each side of the great toe; they seem to be inserted in tendons, and in different places, and are supposed to act as pulleys, increasing power by removing the acting force from the centre of motion.

Having thus generally described the muscles which are necessary for the performance of those varied actions which the foot has to perform, and which are available for all the purposes for which that organ was framed, I would also observe that there is a texture of infinite importance to the muscular system, which assists in giving pliancy and elasticity, and which is an essential part of animal structure; this is the cellular substance. From the lowest grade of vegetable life we trace this tissue, consisting of cells formed of delicate membranes. The first genus of organic products is thus constituted, an aggregation of cells entering into the structure of living beings. It is the medium of communication between the vascular and nervous system, and indeed forms the largest component part of the frame. From this the various tissues are made; and it would seem that it is the function of the living principle to deposit cellular tissue, from which is to be selected such portions as may be necessary to supply the waste of life. As the scale of organized beings ascends so is vascular tissue formed from this, and all the various parts of the body are gradually obtained from this source. Some of the German medical men have of late investigated this subject with peculiar ardour.

London:
PRINTED BY REYNELL AND WEIGHT,
Little Pulteney Street.

4801803R00159

Printed in Great Britain
by Amazon.co.uk, Ltd.,
Marston Gate.